K. SHEHRE BANU

YOGA
NO DRAMA

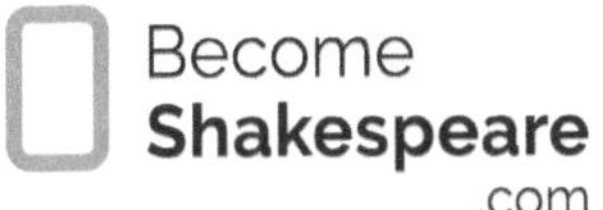

First published in 2020 by

Becomeshakespeare.com

One Point Six Technologies Pvt Ltd.
119-123, 1st Floor, Building J2, B - Wing,
Wadala Truck Terminal,
Wadala East, Mumbai, Maharashtra, India, 400022.
T: +91 85587995915

ISBN - 978-93-90266-22-7

Dedication

To my late father who inspired me to read, as he did, and my late mother who was worried till her last breath about me having a good life. It is because of her that I exist.

Epigraph

*Start where you are, use what you have,
do what you can.*

Table of Contents

6. CAN WE COMPARE APPLES TO APPLES?   154

Yogalates - Module 1   162

7. DO YOU SUFFER FROM SITTING DISEASE?   204

PREFACE

It was 5 PM in the year 2005, when I telephoned my daughter studying in class 2 to inform her that her list of stationery items was packed and would reach her once I reached home. I was happily driving my way back home, thinking how eagerly she would be waiting for me, when suddenly a sumo car hit me! It was purely a hit-and-run case, and I became unplugged.

When I gained consciousness, I was in a hospital amidst strangers who were asking me for my contact number and how this happened. I couldn't piece together what specifically occurred; my memory was blank, and I just had flashbacks of the traumatic event. I had broken my tailbone, injured the cervical soft tissues and damaged the fourth and fifth vertebrae in the lumbar spine. I had bumped my head and injured my forehead and scalp, which had resulted in bleeding under the skin. The doctor had advised total bed rest for an uncertain period and maybe throughout my life. My osteopath had told me that surgery was the only cure for my prolapsed disc. I was shattered and heartbroken.

My physical injuries and mental blocks led me to yoga again – again why?

Because it was yoga that had helped me bring my three wonderful daughters up all alone – single-handedly. I had learned yoga as a hobby somewhere around 1979 and would be extremely joyous when I could turn myself upside down (Shirshasana). After my accident, my chips were down again, and I had nowhere else to go but to the yoga mat. My practice helped me connect to myself and helped me breathe deeply into my physical and emotional scars. Yoga was helping my body repair gently with love, and my spirit was reviving.

It was a healing practice that miraculously got me out of the extreme trauma, and I was filled with joy. My practice isn't a panacea and it didn't eliminate the challenges of life – few days are still hard, and I have my share of struggle in the form of physical pain, bouts of anxiety and depression. However, I have learned to connect my body and mind with my practice, and this provides a stillness to move forward, expand and grow.

As stated by Oprah Winfrey, 'to move forward, choose to give back', I chose to convert this hobby into a profession and decided to teach this divine art as an extension to my counselling and soft skills training.

Bringing up and settling three daughters single-handedly was, and still is, wearing and stressful. Therefore, balancing my career with my yoga training had become hectic. However, it was extremely satisfying, and it taught me to fall graciously in love with my inner self and gradually turned into my passion for life and preventive cure. I eventually took this up as my full-time career.

In this journey of mine, which is nearing two decades, I have come across people of all ages with varied weight loss and health problems, and I am proud and satisfied that I have gained their trust by curing them with the help of Yogabhyasa, increasing my passion for this discipline tenfold.

Take anything of mine away. But my passion – you cannot. And here I write this book with all efforts to make it a simple approach to yoga and Pranayam without any drama i.e. you don't need to be super flexible to practise yoga, you don't need to go to the mountains to practise yoga, you don't need an hour or two on the mat to get results, you don't need to sacrifice your material belongings or become completely vegan or believe in any other such myths that might inhibit you from practising this divine art.

This book should help all women, especially the working professionals who are short of time and are looking out for an adaptable fitness regime. It is for the women who only have 15–20 minutes to stay fit, for the man who wants peace of mind, for the professional who is suffering from back pain or neck and shoulder pains due to long hours of sitting on his chair, for the guy who is looking for a new way to keep fit – as yoga is for everyone and yoga is ageless. No matter who, where and what you are in your life, you can personalise your journey to reach your goal and go back to your mat on your own practice and on your own time. No matter where you are in the world – whether in your backyard, on a holiday, in your living room, in your office or in your bedroom – this book and your mat should help you reach your fitness goals.

Acknowledgments

This book is a result of the immense inspiration and motivation received from my journalist daughter Tasneem Juzar Rampurawala, whose advocacy resulted in penning down my experiences. Writing a book seemed hard to me and it was she who motivated me, believed in me, pushed me, helped me and stood by me in finishing this book, which, after completion is more rewarding than I had ever imagined. My heartfelt. gratitude and sincere thanks to her

Without the help and support from my daughters Tahera and Ruqaiya this book would not exist. Tahera shared most of my home and work-related responsibilities to give me time and space to finish the book. I thank her for her care, understanding, and love.

Ruqaiya, my youngest girl encouraged me every day and every hour to bring this book to life. In spite of her busy schedule, she listened to me patiently and gave me constructive feedback. Thank you Ruqaiya!

A big thanks to everyone who has been a part of this journey, the ones that were a part of my healing process - my mom, my brothers, my sister, and my nephew.

They were the people I could turn to during the years of distress and struggle.

A big thanks to my high school teacher Dolly Shrivastava who not only taught me the noun and the verb but instilled in me the love for the English Language

I am forever indebted to Leah Moses, for her editorial help

I am immensely thankful to everyone on the project management team for helping me so much. Special thanks to the ever patient project managers, Sameer Ambildhok and Shreyas Prathamshetti. Grateful for their ongoing support, their ideas and suggestions helped me polish my manuscript. Thanks to my book cover designer for creating a perfect face for my book.

Thanks to Rohan Patil, the sales advisor from my publishing house - Become Shakespeare; it was he who practically pushed me into publishing this book, by harassing me with his constant calls and messages at any time of the day :). Thanks to him for rescuing the manuscript abandoned in my laptop.

With sincere gratitude, I would like to thank everyone who ever said anything positive to me and has been my teacher. They all have left a positive impact on me.

A huge thanks to all the beautiful souls who have stepped through my door and have graced the mat, and to the souls who still keep stepping through my door and give me energy and love every single day. I am blessed to have you all!

Finally, thanks to Allah, because without him nothing could be done and my Da'i al-Mutlaq Syedna Aali Qadr Mufaddal Saifuddin TUS, who's blessings and prayers made this book possible.

Fit is the goal

Once upon a time, there was a king who was always sick. He was lethargic and tired and fat. As a result, he would lie on his bed all day, getting up just to eat. He assumed he would die soon. Fearing the same, his courtiers summoned various doctors from all over the kingdom. They came and saw the king's condition and desperation and charged a huge amount of fees. They prescribed various medicines that had to be taken daily for months. This was all that the king did – ate medicines, ate food and slept, hoping to get well soon.

One day, a sage came from a distant land. As soon as he heard about the king's condition, he went to see him. When he saw the king, he realised that all that the king needed to do was eat healthily and more importantly EXERCISE (vyayam). He told the king that he would cure him of all his illness, only if he followed his instructions closely and if he would be rewarded half the king's kingdom. The king and his courtiers, desperate to get the king to feel better, decided to agree to his conditions, only if the king's condition improved.

The sage gave the king 10 bagfuls of small round orange tablets and another 10 bagfuls of green square tablets and asked the king to take each of these, three times, everyday. Along with this, he prescribed specific 'vyayam/asanas', which must be followed for the tablets to work. The king reluctantly took the tablets and agreed to perform the 'asanas'.

Days went by, and the king took the tablets and continued exercising. Very soon, he felt much better and fitter. He was happier and wiser. He had never felt better in his life!

After a couple of months, the sage came back to enquire. The king joyously gave him his share of the kingdom and threw a grand ball to welcome the sage. Finally, he asked, "So what were those tablets made of?" The sage replied, "Well, they were nothing but carrots and beans". Saying so, he laughed and left, on his way to his new kingdom.

Isn't this what happens to all of us?

In today's fast-paced life, everyone wants quick fixes to all their problems: We want miraculous cures by putting less effort and we want thrilling and exciting outcomes in a super-duper short timespan. Consequently, we end up getting plugged to the mainstream diet and exercise advice, which keeps screaming:

- "Cardio should be your main workout"

- "Go Paleo or Go Keto"

- "Fad diet, pills and even starvation"

- "Weight loss gadgets"

These fads, which claim weight loss, might help you look skinny, but can spike up your body fat percentage, and you end up being skinny FAT! You may also lose muscles instead of body fat. Ugh, now this causes physical pains, leading to emotional agony, and the story goes on.

The evidence says that many exercise fads have come and gone, offering short-term solutions to long-term problems. However, what remained with us is the 5000-year-old practice of yoga. Regardless of yoga being the black horse in the race of weight loss, this book shall help you gain clarity on various myths such as:

- Yoga is too gentle or mild for weight loss.

- Weight loss happens slowly with yoga – you have to bust your butt in the gym to get results faster!

- Yoga is for women who are young, flexible and slender.

- Yoga needs an hour or more, and I am busy.

'The less we respond to drama, the more peaceful our life becomes', and this is what the book is basically written for – ignore the myths and forget the drama. Simply understand the fact that yoga, when fused with pilates and cardio, not only aids in calorie burning but also builds stamina, tones and sculpts the body, strengthens the core, de-stresses and detoxifies.

This book will guide you on how to alert your body and alter its structure by consistently practising yoga everyday for six months. Body sculpting is made possible with yoga as it can reverse even genetic predispositions. How? There are specific asanas (which work internally) that can be focussed on the problem areas. The asanas also work on the hormonal imbalances and digestive system, thus bringing about an inner balance and automatically aids in weight loss.

The sequences of asanas mentioned in the chapter on flexibility work out those muscles that are normally not used much, including stretching and lengthening them in an overall safe and effective manner. So even if you are above 40 years of age (the age where we gradually lose our flexibility) and start practising yoga consistently, your practice shall help you regain the lost flexibility and balance, caused by the effects of being over 40.

Office goers struggle to find time to work out, as work specifically gets in the way of working out. The chapter on Surya Namaskars should help them as it explains how this gracefully linked sequence of asanas can be a complete body workout for fitness and weight loss in a limited time span with additional benefits like gaining confidence, stamina, vitality, ingenuity and increased mental and instinctive abilities. To make it more cardio-intensive, you can include in your session a few cardio yoga drills from the chapter number 5 - 'Cardio Yoga', and get the best of both worlds.

The chapter on cardio yoga will prove to be a boon for people who feel that Surya Namaskars are boring and monotonous and for people who have less time when it comes to fitness. Cardio plays the role of a king when it comes to fat burning, and yoga helps in maintaining muscle tone, stimulates the endocrine system, regulates the metabolic rate, decreases the stress levels and forbids weight gain.

It is a strenuous type of a fusion of yoga and cardio, which keeps you moving with challenging poses and sequences and maximizes calorie burn.

The chapter on yogalates demonstrates how yoga and pilates, when fused together, fires up the core, tones muscles, stimulates the internal organs and helps in the detoxification of the body.

The chapter on sitting disease deals with how sitting has become the new smoking and how to get rid of this disease and get moving by doing simple yoga asanas.

This is not the first book on yoga and its immense benefits; you will find thousands of such books. However, here in this book, I have tried to show how easy it is to build your fitness regime into your working day and how to integrate yoga into your daily routine – without drama – without feeling guilty of using up your valuable time.

This book has been written with a mission: ANYONE with ANY body type, at ANY age, with ANY level of fitness can (and should) do yoga – because it's no more a drama, it's no more boring and it's no more a slow-paced workout! We have taken care of all these by integrating yoga with pilates, cardio and power yoga.

Take out your mats and start where you are and enjoy the journey!

CHAPTER 1

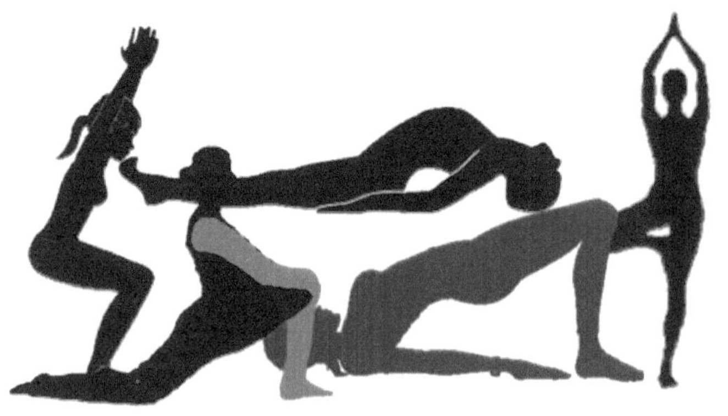

1. STRETCH, NOT STRESS!

"But I am inflexible and cannot stretch," said Reena.

"Reena, this is not for the 'flexible', but for the willing. Are you willing to stretch?" asked her trainer.

The rest of the participants were deeply engrossed in their yogic pose. Reena looked at them apprehensively.

"I think I am willing, but a little scared that I might tear my muscles or break my bones," replied Reena hesitantly.

The trainer smiled back saying, "Don't worry! Yogis who practice bending don't break."

The popular yoga myth is, "Can I do yoga as I am not flexible?" It's like saying, "Can I take a bath, even though I am so dirty?" The answer is you need not be flexible before you set your foot on your mat. Flexibility is never a prerequisite on a yoga mat. Every being is born flexible, and that is why as infants we easily put our toes in our mouth. The saying, "If you don't use it, you lose it" applies to flexibility too... read on.

In this world, where there is a race for burning fat/ improve cardiovascular endurance/build strength, what limps along as an afterthought is "flexibility training" – an important component of fitness, which the Oxford English Dictionary defines as "the quality of bending easily, without breaking." Although it is a must in our daily exercise routine, it is not done so, maybe because of a compressed workout schedule in today's busy world.

Why flexibility training?

Basically to aid freedom of movement with no more worries when you bend down to tie your shoelace, scratch your back or look back as you drive and also to minimize energy usage during physical activity, lessen chances of injury by reducing muscle tightness, balancing tissue extensibility and reducing joint degeneration. Not forgetting the age-related 'flexibility crisis', it becomes a boon for 40+ age groups!

How to overcome time constraints?

I cannot fit it in my regular fitness workouts. If this is so, then I suggest that you choose a workout such as a yogalates workout, a cardio yoga workout or a hot yoga workout, where flexibility goes hand in hand with the other essentials such as strength training, cardiovascular endurance, etc., which come as a BONUS! The bends and twists work on your body and convert you into a HUMAN PRETZEL, just as the quote says, "Yogi's don't break they bend."

Flexibility depends on various factors such as age, gender, sedentary lifestyle, to some extent the size of the body and also practising excessive exercise of the same type. The development of your muscles also decides how flexible you are. Overdeveloped muscles (in certain sports) almost always reduce flexibility. If some muscles are weak (due to underuse), it leads to a drop in the flexibility level too.

A study was conducted by the University of Wisconsin on 34 healthy women of age approximately 33 years, who were divided into two groups– a yoga group, and a non-yoga control group. The yoga group had to do 55 minutes of yogabhyasa thrice a week, which came up to 21 classes in all. The study concluded that the yoga group's average flexibility improved from 13% to 35%, and gains were significant. Flexibility changes were seen in the entire body, shoulder girdle, twisting, bending, reaching, good lower back flexibility, etc. This, I think, has a very good carryover to everyday life.

I hope by now it's clear that flexibility is the modern-day efficacy that everybody needs and wants. But flexibility comes with a cost! And what is that? Well, it is incorporating a regular fitness workout that targets the main factors of fitness: cardio, muscle strength and flexibility.

Flexibility training involves asanas that focus on the major muscle–tendon groups of the shoulder, chest, neck, trunk, lower back, hips, hamstrings, quadriceps and ankles Mentioned below are a few asanas and sequences that focus primarily on flexibility gain.

Forward bending asanas

Forward bends open up the hips, pelvis, glutes, inner thigh muscles, calf muscles and lower back. They work best to improve flexibility in the hamstrings.

If the purpose is to stretch and not stress, then it is important we keep in mind a few points before we get into a forward bend:

- Do not round your spine just to get deeper into a pose.

- Keep your neck and spine long and take your chest forward to the thighs.

- Bend from your hips and tilt your pelvis down and do not use your back muscles for the forward fall.

- If your hamstrings (inner thigh muscles) are tight, then contract your quads (upper thigh muscles) to release your hamstrings.

- Expand your chest and pull your shoulder blades down your spine.

- Practise mindfully, and understand the point where you can feel mild tension and not a feeling of pain.

A word of caution: Do not ever get pulled or pushed too far into a forward bend as it can injure your spinal disks and ligaments.

Listed below are the most effective forward bending poses:

Uttanasana/standing head to knee pose and ardha uttanasana/standing half forward bend pose (for beginners):

Uttanasana:

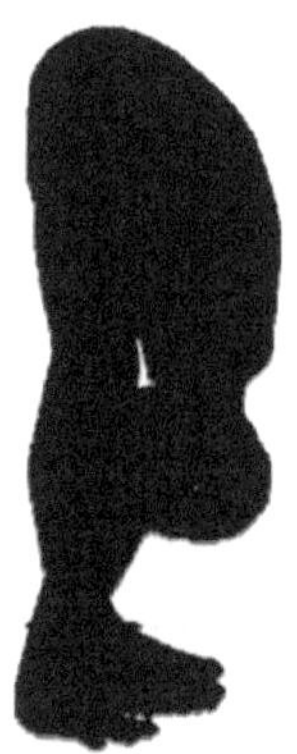

1. Stand in tadasana.

   What is tadasana? It is a standing pose with a straight back and shoulders away from the ears (by rotating the shoulders outwards).

2. Open the chest by drawing the shoulder blades down towards the spine.

3. Distribute weight equally on the corners of your feet.

4. Pause for 2 counts in tadasana, and then slowly bend down from your hips, keeping them in line with your heels.

5. As you bend, engage your core, elongate your neck in line with your spine and bring your chest to your thighs.

6. The crown of your head faces the mat.

7. Reach for your ankles or your shin, or cup your fingers and place the tips on the mat.

8. Alternatively, bend your knees or place your hands on blocks to help reach the ground.

9. You can bend your knees slightly and hold onto your shins to lessen the stretch.

10. Practise normal breathing in this pose.

Ardha uttanasana:

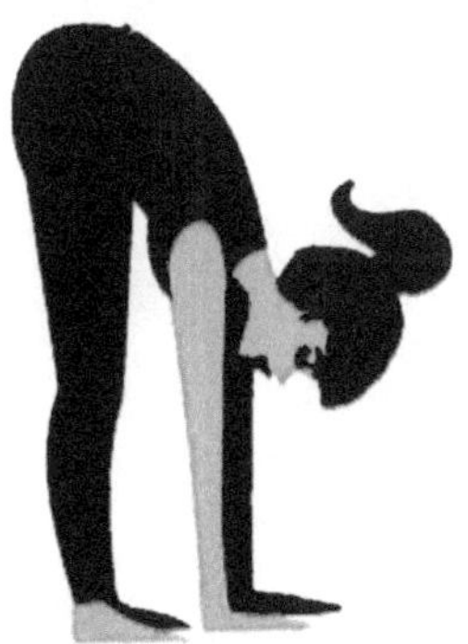

Points 1 to 5 are the same as in UTTANASANA

6. As you bend down from your hips, lift up from your heart.

7. Bend till your torso is parallel to the mat.

8. Reach the mat or your toes.

9. Bend a little more if you cannot reach the mat.

10. You can also place your hands on a block to help reach the mat.

11. Practise normal breathing in this pose.

Parsvottanasana/pyramid pose:

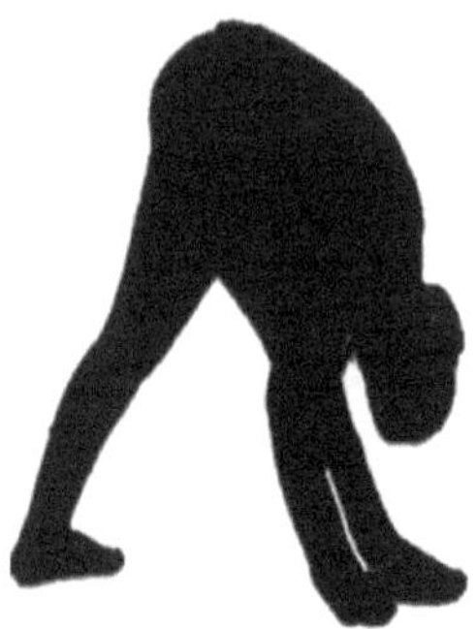

1. Stand in tadasana.

2. Step your left foot behind yourself, with your toes turning out at 45° angle.

3. Align your heels in line.

4. Gradually bend from your hips and extend your torso over your right leg.

5. Keep your spine long and neck neutral.

6. Bring your belly towards your thigh.

7. You can either fold your arms behind or bring them down on the mat beside your right foot.

8. Practise normal breathing in this pose.

Navasana/Full boat pose:

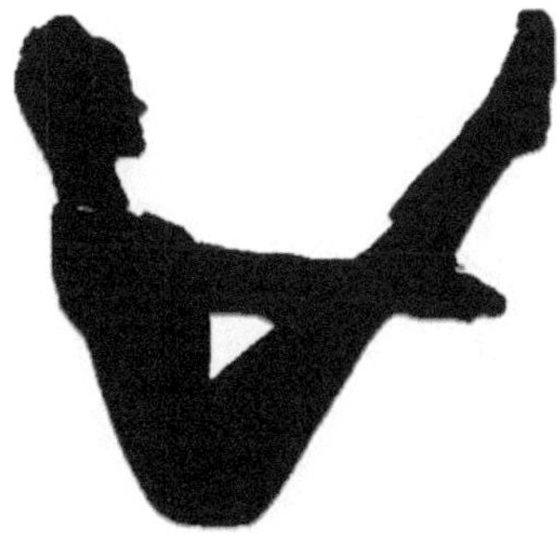

Full boat pose:

1. You can either begin by sitting in staff pose or sitting with your knees bent and feet flat on the floor. Rest your hands beside your hips with palms flat on the mat.

2. Engage your core, keep your spine straight, lean back a little, lift your feet up and bring your shins parallel to the mat.

3. Open your chest, draw your lower back in, leng then your torso, straighten your legs at a 45⁰ angle with the mat and bring your body in a V shape.

4. Simultaneously raise and extend your arms forward, in line with your shoulder and palms facing each other.

5. Gaze forward and keep your hands and feet active.

6. Practise normal breathing in this pose.

Ardha navasana/Half boat pose (for beginners):

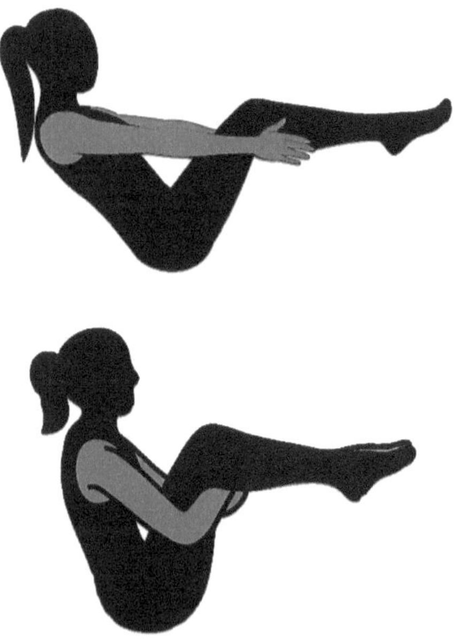

1. Begin by sitting with your knees bent and feet flat on the floor. Rest your hands beside your hips with your palms flat on the mat.

2. Lift your legs so that the lower leg is parallel to the mat and arms reach forward, parallel to the mat.

3. For additional support, you can hold the back of the thighs. Gently pull your thighs further towards your abs and knees towards your chest to challenge your core strength and stability.

Virabhadrasana 3/Warrior 3 pose:

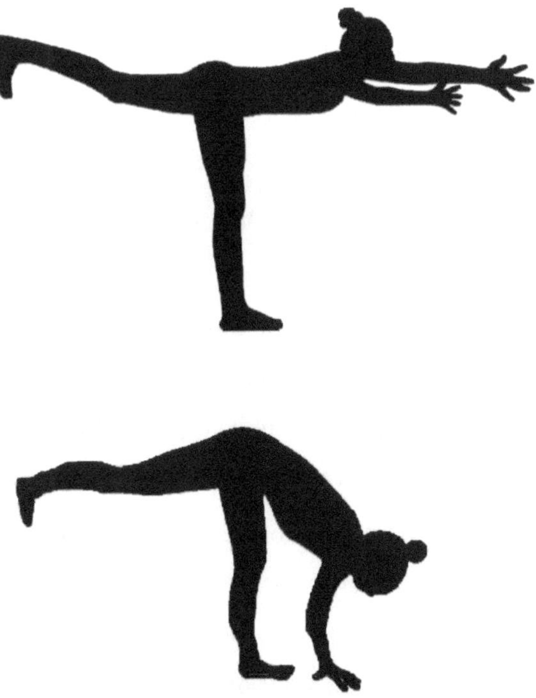

1. Begin from tadasana, standing with your legs hip-distance apart and arms at your side.

2. Extend your left foot backward and pivot it around 45° inwards.

3. Your right foot should be perpendicular to the top of the mat with your toes pointing forward.

4. Turn your pelvis and torso towards your right toes.

5. Slowly lift up your left leg, drawing your tummy to your spine.

6. Lower your torso and bring your body parallel to the ground.

7. Simultaneously extend arms forward. Try to keep your arms straight and engaged.

8. Micro-bend the right knee.

9. Flex the lifted foot and actively engage it. Push through the heel as though you are pushing the wall.

10. Create length through your neck by gazing ahead of you downwards (to the top of the mat).

11. Keep your spine long and square your hips evenly to the ground.

12. If you are a beginner, you can try this pose by keeping both your arms on the mat (as shown

in the picture), or place your palms on two blocks kept on the mat beside both your feet.

13. You can even take the support of the wall, by placing the foot of the flying leg flat on the wall.

14. You can even avoid taking the lifted leg high.

15. Keep the standing leg strong and engage your hip muscles (squeeze your hip and thigh muscles for balance).

16. Engage your whole core, your side waist (obliques), your lower abdomen and your back muscles.

17. Practise normal breathing in this pose.

Malasana/Garland pose/Yogic low squat:

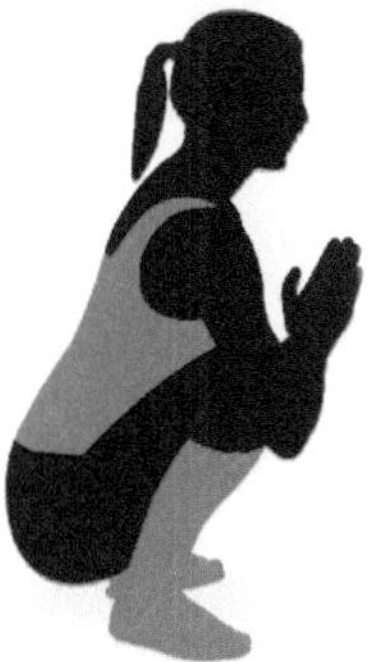

1. Begin in tadasana.

2. Place your legs outside of your hips and point your toes slightly out.

3. Slowly press down and drop your hips as far down as comfortable.

4. You can take support by placing your palms on the mat near your toes.

5. See to it that your knees point in the direction of your toes. If your hips are tight, your knees might turn inwards. Therefore, listen to your body and do not try to exceed your limits.

6. If your heels lift up, it is fine. However, if you can, try to keep them down, but do not force them.

7. Once down and comfortable, press your palms together near your chest.

8. Keep lengthening your spine.

9. Widen your knees with your elbows to open up your hips more.

10. If your heels are close to touching the mat, widen your stance to see if they touch.

11. If not, take a towel or a rolled-up mat and place it under your heels.

12. Now open up your ankles and hips and relax.

13. As there is no one-size-fits-all squat, keep adjusting your stance width or your elbow placement until you are comfortable in the pose.

14. Practise normal breathing in this pose.

15. To come out of the pose, place your hands on the mat near your toes and slowly rise up to standing forward bend and then to tadasana.

Janu sirsasana/Head-to-knee forward bend pose:

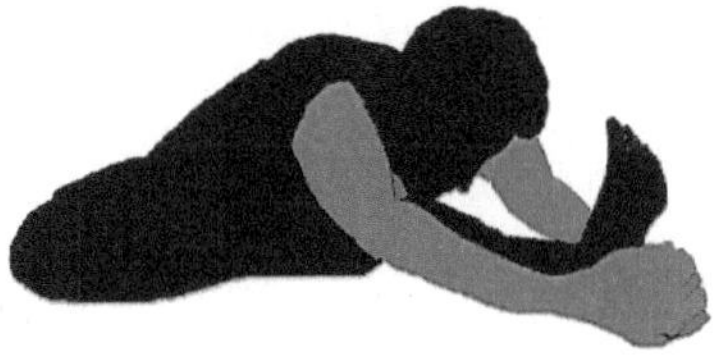

1. Begin seated in long sitting, with your spine straight and arms beside your hips.

2. Widen your legs until they are perpendicular to each other.

3. Fold your right leg, bringing the sole of your right foot to meet your left inner thigh.

4. Your right heel should touch your left groin. Your right knees, right leg and the outer edge of your right foot should rest on the floor. Relax the bent right knee towards the floor.

5. Gently bend forward from your hips, extend your arms and grasp your left foot. If you cannot reach

your foot, you can grasp the ankle, calves or shin of the left leg.

6. Elongate your spine and lengthen your neck.

7. If possible, lower your elbows on the floor and lower your chest and your face towards your left leg.

8. Repeat the same with the other leg.

9. Practise normal breathing in this pose.

Uttana shishosana/Extended puppy pose:

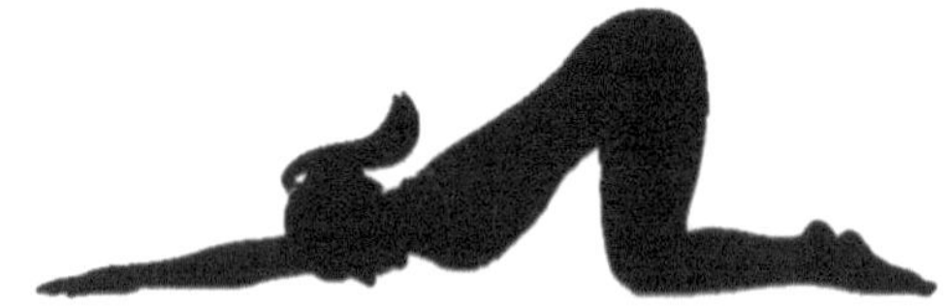

1. Begin on all fours.

2. Stack your shoulders, elbows, and wrists. Similarly, stack your hips and knees.

3. Walk your arms forward and drop your chest on the mat.

4. Your hips should remain over the knees.

5. Your arms should be shoulder-width apart.

6. Pull your navel up and push your hips back.

7. Gently draw your forehead on the mat (do not force yourself. Draw it down till body permits).

8. Relax your neck and keep your shoulders soft.

9. If possible, you can extend your arms a little further and lay your chest on the mat too. This should give you an intense stretch in your spine.

10. To come out of the pose, you can either power your hips down and get into makarasana, or you can walk your hands in and lift up your body and stand on your knees.

11. Practise normal breathing in this pose.

Upavistha konasana/Seated wide-angle forward bend pose:

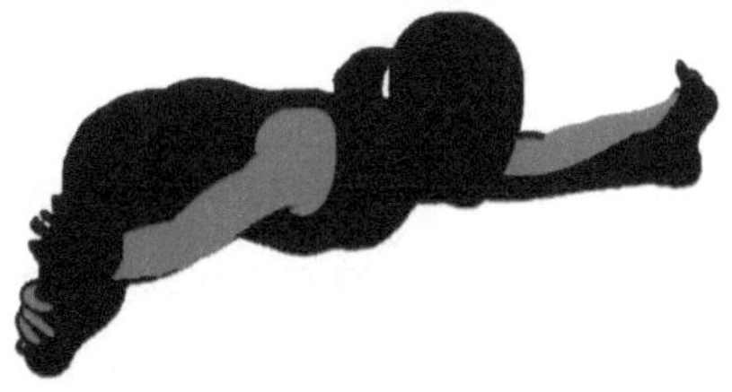

1. Sit in long sitting with your legs wide. Initially, your legs should be stretched at 90 degrees angle.

2. Extend your arms forward with your palms facing down and on the mat.

3. Bend forward, bring your pelvis down, and extend your legs a little more – 10 degrees to 20 degrees more.

4. Press your thigh bones into the ground and walk hand forward. Simultaneously keep extending your legs.

5. Your toes should be flexed and pointing inwards towards you.

6. Keep your neck long and spine straight.

7. There are possibilities of your spine curving if you hurry to get deeper in the pose. Therefore, do not hurry, and remember that it is the process that is more important.

8. Keep stretching until your back remains straight and is comfortable.

9. If depth in the pose matters to you and gives you satisfaction, then you can place a folded blanket under your sit bones. This helps in the tipping of the pelvis.

10. A blanket under your knees provides extra support.

11. You can also support your spine by sitting against a wall.

12. Practise normal breathing in this pose.

13. To come out of the pose, lift your torso up, bring your arms back to the sides of your body and bring your knees together.

Prasirita padottanasana/ Standing wide-legged forward bend pose:

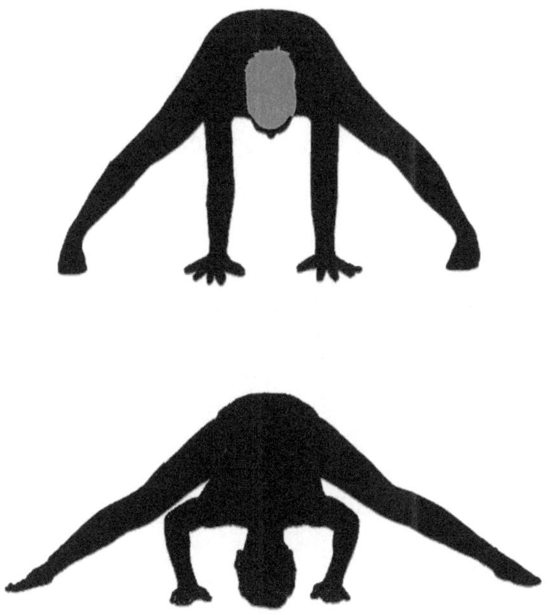

1. Stand in tadasana.

2. Widen your legs with your toes pointing slightly inwards (to protect your knees).

3. Bring your arms to your hips, expand your chest and fold forward at the hips.

4. Release your hands from your hips and simultaneously bring them down as you bend down. Place them down on the mat, shoulder-width apart, with your palms flat on the mat.

5. Adjust your body and see to it that your hips are above your ankles.

6. Keep your neck long and spine neutral.

7. The moment you feel discomfort in your back, bend your knees and go only as far as your body permits.

8. If possible, bend your arms from your elbows and try to reach your head to the mat. Keeping your head on the mat adds up to support and balance.

9. You can use a bolster or a block or a blanket to place your head.

10. Practise normal breathing in this pose.

11. To come out of the pose, twist your torso upright by engaging your leg muscles and pressing your feet slightly into the mat.

Ananda balasana/happy baby pose:

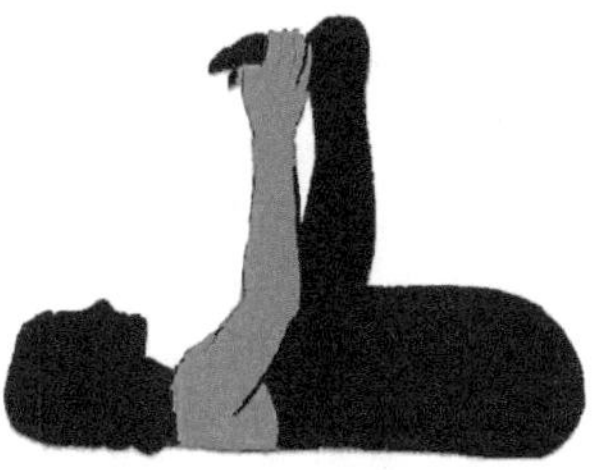

1. Lie on your back with a neutral spine position.

2. Bring your knees to your chest and raise your calves and feet up, with your hips staying down.

3. Flex your feet and let the soles of your feet face the roof.

4. Your legs should be parallel to each other.

5. Your shoulders should stay on the mat and should not rise up.

6. Extend your arms up to the outside of your foot and wrap your fingers on the arch of your feet. Gently pull your feet down so that the knees come closer to your chest.

7. Relax your back, shoulder and neck – all in contact with the mat. Soften your hips and be a happy baby.

8. If you cannot reach the foot, hold your shin or ankles.

9. Practise normal breathing in this pose.

10. To come out of the pose, release your arms, straighten your legs and rest in shavasana.

Adho mukha svanasana/downward facing dog:

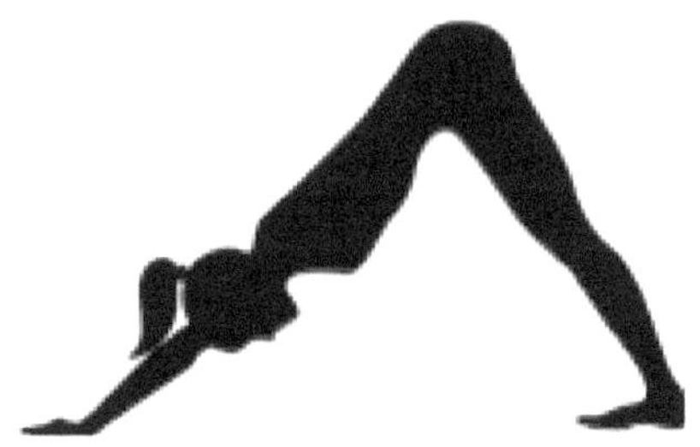

1. Begin in tadasana.

2. Open your palms, bend your knees and lower your body straight down to half lift.

3. Place your palms or fingertips on the mat beside your feet and spread your fingers wide.

4. Externally rotate your shoulders and spread your shoulder blades wide.

5. Let your arms be wide at shoulder distance.

6. Straighten your legs, lower your heels towards the mat, lift your hips up, coming into an upside-down "V" shape.

7. Your body might not permit your heels to touch the mat. This is fine, and therefore, do not force yourself.

8. Relax your head between your arms, push your body in and look inwards towards your knees.

9. Practise normal breathing and stay in the pose for 10 to 20 seconds.

10. Once you are comfortable with this, proceed to the next exercise.

Ek pada svanasana/one-legged dog (for the intermediate practitioners):

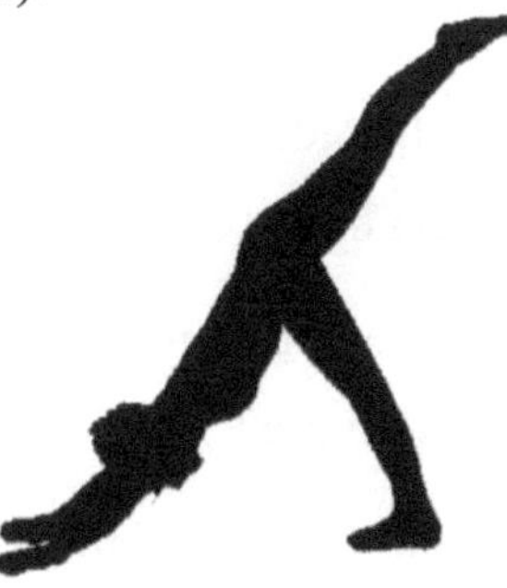

1. From the downward-facing dog position, raise your right foot up to the roof and root the left foot into the mat.

2. Lengthen your spine, square your hips and square your shoulders.

3. Rotate your shoulder blades inwards and reach your head to the mat.

4. Your arms should be wide at shoulder distance.

5. Keep gazing at the back.

6. Repeat with the other leg.

7. Practise normal breathing in this pose.

The backward bending asanas:

These asanas are excellent for strengthening the back and restoring the natural flexibility of the spine. The spine becomes strong and super flexible.

The backbend asanas tone the entire core and increase the range of motion of the abdominal region.

As they lengthen the body, they ease the tight muscles and make you feel limber.

Back-bending asanas can be challenging if you are just starting out your practice. This is because, we spend the major part of our day in an unsupported forward bend. As a result, there could be stiffness in your neck, shoulders and back muscles.

Here are few simple tips for a safe backbend:

- Keep your neck long.

- Open your chest and open your hip flexors.

- Keep elongating your spine.

- Relax your shoulder.

- Keep your core engaged and try to arch your entire spine.

There are a few great backbends that even a beginner can practice safely.

Bhujangasana/Upward facing dog pose:

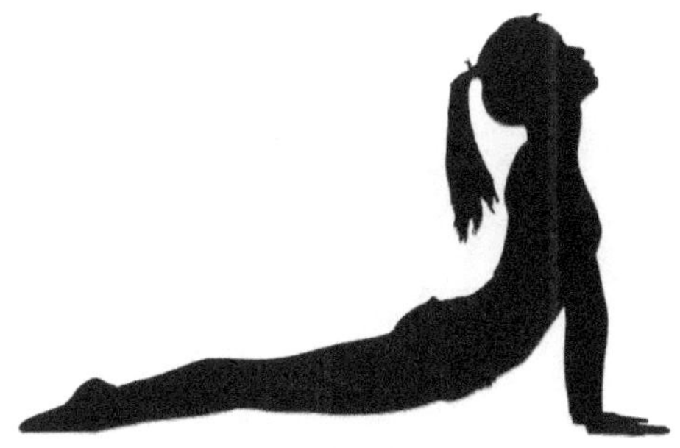

1. Begin with lying on the abdomen.

2. Your Legs should be stretched with your knees and front of your feet touching the mat.

3. Your chin should be on the mat.

4. Bring your palms beside your armpits.

5. Pressing the hips on the mat, gently raise your chest up.

6. Press your shoulders down and back, and arch your spine evenly.

7. Bend backward as much as you can and gaze up.

8. Your hips have to remain planted onto the mat and your navel off the mat.

9. To come out of the pose, bend your arms and lower your chest, shoulders and forehead.

Setu bandhasana/Bridge pose:

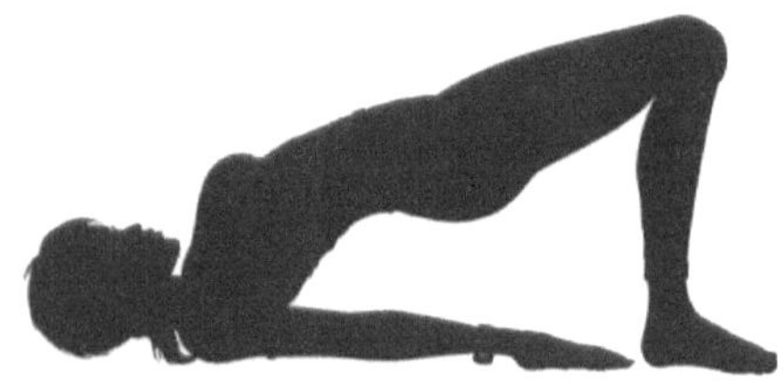

1. Begin in a supine position.

2. Fold your legs at the knees, with your feet flat on the mat and hip-distance away.

3. Stack your knees and heels.

4. Arms are straight beside your body with your palms facing down.

5. Bring your feet close to your buttocks.

6. Broaden your collar bones, and lift your chest and buttocks up, away from the floor.

7. Gently press the centre of your head onto the mat.

8. Squeeze your buttocks and keep your lower back safe.

9. Slowly move your chin away from your chest, so that there is a slight gap between your neck and the mat.

10. Drive your hip more up and forward.

11. The inner edges of the feet should be parallel to each other.

12. Gaze up.

Matsyasana/Fish pose:

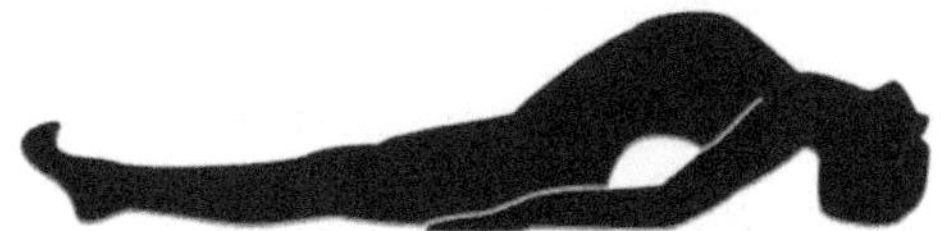

1. Begin in a supine pose.

2. Your arms should rest beside your sides and your legs should be extended and close to each other, with your palms facing down.

3. Bring your arms under your hips, press your elbows lightly and raise your chest and head off the mat.

4. Gently bring the crown of your head on the mat, keeping your toes pointed.

5. Ensure that there is no pressure on your head and neck.

6. To come out of the pose, release your torso and head to the mat.

Salabhasana/Locust pose:

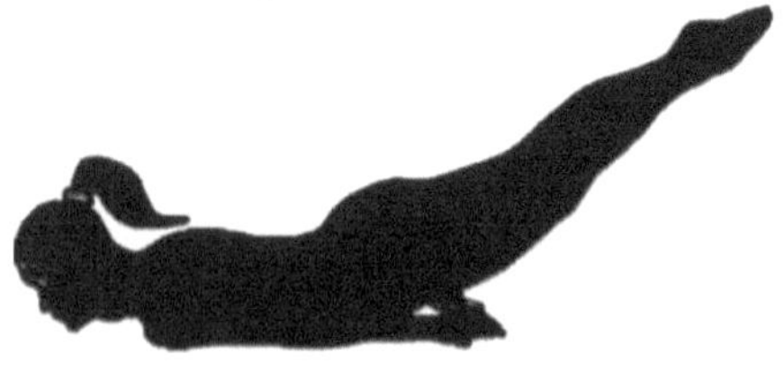

1. Begin in the prone pose (lie on your stomach).

2. Your arms should be beside your sides, with your palms facing up.

3. Rest your forehead on the floor.

4. Slide your palms under your thighs.

5. Lift up your head, chest and legs away from the mat. Your knees should not bend.

6. Your stomach, pelvis and lower ribs should remain on the mat.

7. Firming your buttocks and energizing your legs, lengthen your back legs. Activate your toes.

8. Gaze forward or slightly upward.

9. Keep your neck long and the base of the skull lifted.

10. To come out of the pose, bring your head down and rest your chin. Lower your legs down and relax your arms.

Dhanurasana/Bow pose:

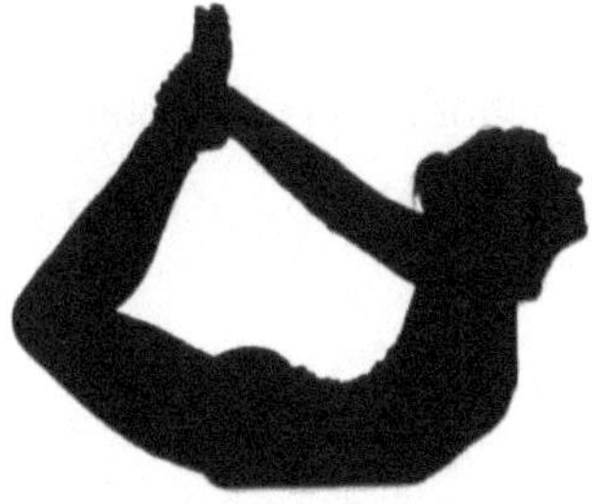

1. Begin in the prone pose.

2. Your knees should be hip-distance apart.

3. Lift your heart forward and up, and lift your head and chest off the mat.

4. Fold your knees.

5. Drawing the shoulder blades towards each other, reach your arms behind and grab your ankles with the respective arms. Pull your heels closer to your hips, with your arms remaining straight.

6. Keep your knees in line with your hips and do not spread them further apart.

7. Tightening your thighs, raise the knees high up above the mat.

8. Pushing your knees back and up, raise your pelvis off the mat too.

9. The weight of your body should be onto your abdomen and navel.

10. To come out of the pose, gently release your ankles and lower torso down and bring your legs down.

Ustrasana/Camel pose:

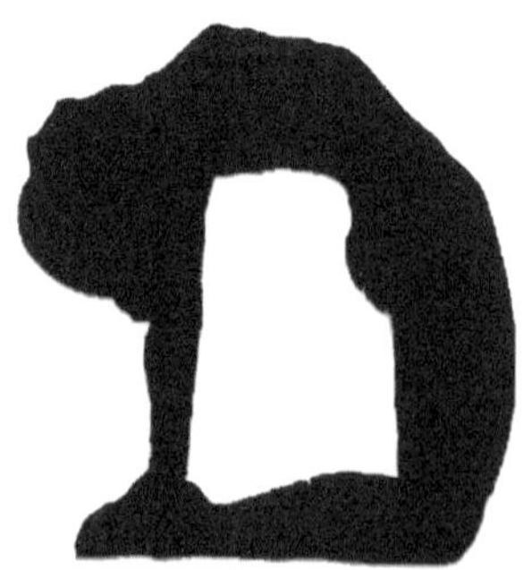

1. Begin by standing on your knees, with your knees hip-distance apart.

2. Stack your hips over your knees by pushing them forward.

3. Your feet should be hip-distance apart, with your toes flat on mat and the front of your feet pressing the mat lightly. Beginners can start with keeping your feet on your toes.

4. Your thighs should be parallel to each other. Similarly, your shins should remain parallel to each other and pressed on the mat.

5. Hold the sides of your hips, engage your thighs, roll your shoulders, expand your chest and arch yourself up, back and down.

6. Rotating your shoulders back, reach for your heels, or, if possible, your respective soles. If you cannot reach your heels, then reach for your shins or calves.

7. Your hips should remain right above the your knees.

8. Let your head fall back without any force. Keep your neck relaxed and your shoulders soft.

9. Do not curl your spine but keep it long.

10. Gaze at the roof.

11. To come out of the pose, release your hands and put them back on your hips.

12. Curl back up – your belly, your torso and finally your head.

Anjaneyasana/Crescent moon/Low lunge backbend:

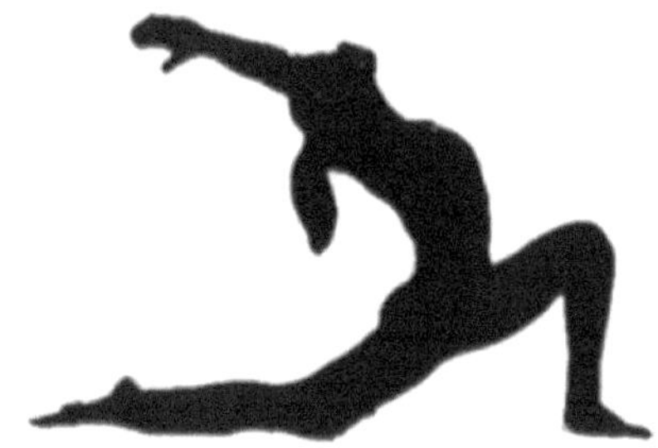

1. Begin in the downward dog pose or in half lift.

2. From the downward dog pose, step your right foot forward between your palms.

3. Lower your left knee onto the mat, and also place the top of your left foot on the mat.

4. Adjust your left leg till your right knee is over the heel.

5. Lifting your torso up, raise your arms up and overhead.

6. Gently stretch your head back and look at your hands, keeping your neck long and relaxed.

7. To come out of the pose, bring your arms down and palms beside your right foot. Move your right foot back and return to the downward dog pose.

8. Repeat the same with the other leg.

The twisting asanas:

These enable detoxification and regeneration of scar tissues that are causing stiffness and inhibiting flexibility. This is procured by cutting off the blood supply to organs and muscles and then supplying them with a fresh supply of blood.

Parivritta trikonasana/Revolved triangle pose:

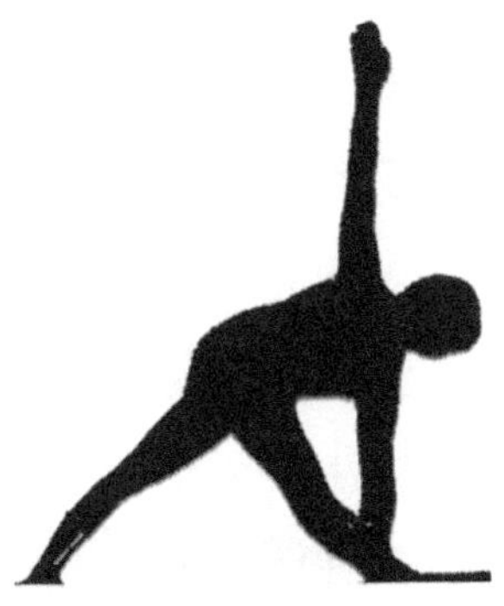

1. Begin in tadasana.

2. Spread your legs wide apart and turn the right foot such that it is perpendicular to the front of the mat. Both your heels should be in a line and the heel of the back foot should be pointing back.

3. Extend your arms sideways in line with your shoulders and parallel to the floor with your palms facing downwards.

4. Turn your head towards the right side, reach forward to lengthen, raise the right arm up and gently twist your torso and head – from the waist, towards your right.

5. Maintain stability in your legs, bring your left hand down and put your left palm on the mat beside your right foot or beyond your right foot on the outer side of your foot. If you cannot reach the mat with your palm, you can cup your left-hand finger.

6. The sides of your torso should be in line and parallel to your right leg.

7. Tuck in your belly, relax and contract your shoulders and open your chest.

8. Gaze at the roof or your right-hand thumb.

9. Repeat with the other leg.

10. To come out of the pose, balance lightly on your left heel, lift up your left hand and rotate your torso back to tadasana.

Utthita parsvakonasana/Revolved side angle:

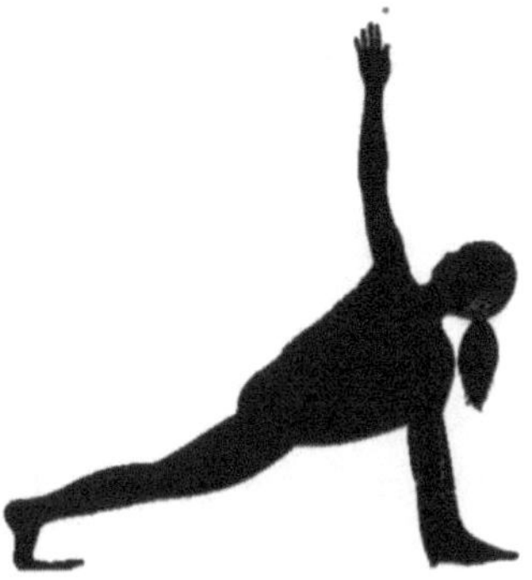

1. Begin in the downward dog pose or tadasana.

2. If you begin in the downward dog pose, then extend your right leg forward and place it in between your palms.

3. Your right knee should be stacked over your right ankle or slightly behind. Your right thigh should make a 90° angle with your right calf, parallel to the mat.

4. You will be in a high lunge position, wherein both your heels are in line with each other. Extend your left leg straight behind and engage your left thigh muscles.

5. Bring your left palm to the outer side of your right foot, twist your torso and your head towards the right side and lift up your right arm upwards besides your right ear. Your right arm should be perpendicular to your right side.

6. Press your left hand gently into the mat such that the back of your left armpit is against the outside of your right knee. Lengthen the right side of your body all the way from your right foot to your right fingertips.

7. Keep your shoulders soft.

8. Expand your chest and pull it slightly backwards such that your chest, hips, and right leg all stay in one line.

9. To come out of the pose, bring your right hand down and place your palm beside the outside of your foot.

10. Go back to downward dog pose and repeat on the other side.

Ardha matsyendrasana/Seated spinal twist:

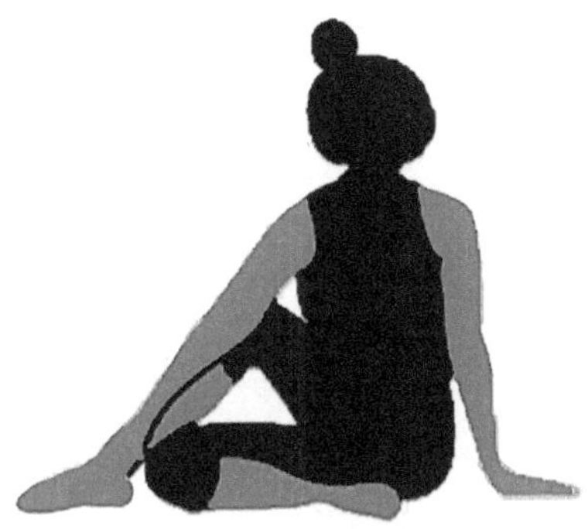

1. Begin in the long sitting pose.

2. Fold your right leg and bring your right ankle close to your left buttocks.

3. Lift up your left hip, hold your right ankle and pull your right foot close to your left hip such that your right heel touches your left hip.

4. The outside edge of your right foot, your ankle and your pinky toe should be pressed into the mat.

5. Fold your left leg, hold your left foot and bring it next to the outside of your right thigh and place it in such a way that your left shin remains perpendicular to the mat.

6. Your torso should be straight with your chin raised up.

7. Your right arm should be straight beside your hip with your palm facing downwards and fingertips facing forward.

8. Twist from your navel towards the left side.

9. Bring your right arm towards the left and twist more to place your right upper arm in front of the outside of your left knee. If possible, press your right armpit into your left knee.

10. Straightening your right arm, slightly try and grab your left ankle.

11. Expand your chest, swing your left arm behind your back and roll over your middle back with your palms facing out and fingertips over your right waist.

12. Turn your head towards the left and gaze over your left shoulder.

13. Breathe normally, keep your shoulders and neck relaxed and keep twisting your torso more inch by inch.

14. To come out of the pose, release your right arm, unfold your left arm and untwist.

15. Repeat the same on the other side.

Parivrtta anjaneyāsana/Crescent twist:

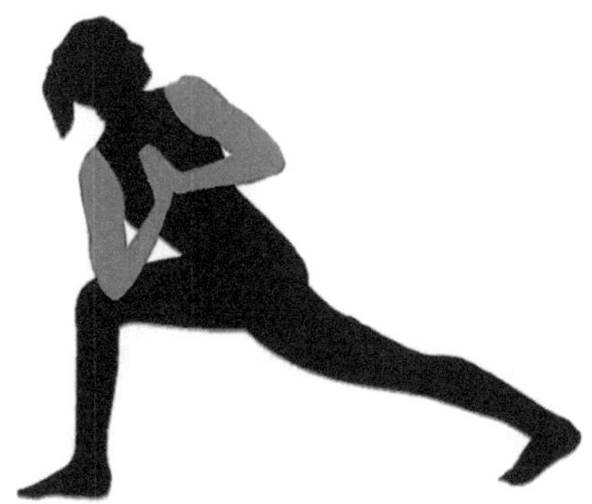

1. Begin in the crescent pose, with your right leg forward. Your palms should be together at your heart centre.

2. Gently twist towards your right side, place your left tricep on your right thigh first and then snuggle your left elbow outside your right knee.

3. Bring your torso as close as possible to your leg.

4. Keep squaring your hips by twisting your torso instead of your hips.

5. Another way to do this pose is to snuggle your left armpit outside your right knee and place your left fingers on the mat.

6. Extend your right arm up and gaze up at the roof.

7. To come out of the pose, untwist and rise back to the crescent or to the downward-facing dog pose.

8. Repeat on the other side.

Again, I repeat, stretch and never stress your joints, muscles or ligaments. You can initially use props such as straps, blocks and bolsters, as these tools support your body and stretch the muscles by helping you find better length in each posture. You can also use the wall as your support.

If practising has to be made dynamic and interesting, you can sequence these asanas and repeat the sequence for 2 to 3 rounds.

I have compiled them into 4 sequences, which include all the above asanas:

Sequence-1	Sequence-2	Sequence-3	Sequence-4
1. Mountain pose	1. Mountain pose	1.Mountain Pose	1. Child pose
2. Standing head-to-knee pose	2. Warrior 3 (right leg)	2. Standing head-to-knee pose	2. Camel pose

3. Downward-facing dog pose	3. Pyramid pose (left leg forward)	3.Garland pose	3. On fours
4. One-legged dog pose with right leg	4. One-legged down dog pose (raising the left leg up)	4. Boat	4. Extended puppy pose
5. High lunge with the right leg in front	5.Ardh uttanasana (bringing left leg forward)	5.Wide-angle seated forward bend pose	5. Cobra pose
6. Crescent twist	6. Mountain pose	6. Seated spinal twist (both sides)	6. Locust pose
7. Plank	7. Repeat with the other leg (step 2 to 5)	7. (Lie down on your back) happy baby pose	7. Bow pose

8. Cobra pose	8. Gently get into Malasana pose	Shavasana	8. Child pose
9. Downward dog pose – repeat from step 3	9. Seated forward bend		9. Long sitting pose, on your back and bridge pose
10. Standing wide-legged forward bend	10. Boat pose		10. Shavasana
11. Makarasana	11. On your back and bridge pose		
	12. Rise up for a spinal twist on the right side.		

	13. Then a spinal twist on the left side.		
	13. Shavasana		

These are easy, simple and quick and can be practised at home. They do not require any equipment.

You can incorporate these sequences into your exercise routines or practise them separately.

Stay in each pose for a minimum of 3 counts initially, gradually increasing it to 8 counts keeping in mind your personal rhythm.

Practice mindfully with normal breathing.

How long does it take to gain flexibility? I have been asked this question by almost all the candidates when they come for inquiry. The answer is a simple honest one and i.e. you give me your 10 to 15 minutes every day, and I will help you make it twofold in one month. The repetition of asanas creates flexibility and therefore the body becomes supple, the transition from one pose to the other becomes simpler and you can also get into the depth of the poses.

You simply have to add these stretches after every class. In case you can't fit them into your schedule, you could do the following:

- You can do them immediately after a shower or

- Before you get out of bed in the morning or

- After an afternoon nap or

- Take out 10 to 15 minutes during your work hours in the office.

To get rid of your flexibility crisis, maintain a consistent practice and you will see amazing results.

Why?

Because we are all naturally flexible and we have just lost it...don't believe me? Then spend some time with kids under 6 years and you'll agree to the fact that they are all 'born yogis.'

The FITT of flexibility

Frequency:

Flexibility exercises are ideal after every workout because as the muscles are warm, they ease the flexibility training and make it comfortable. If you want to improve flexibility at a faster rate, and if you are young, then practise these asanas at least twice a day for 10–15 minutes. Flexibility training 2–3 times per week could be effective, but greater gain in the range of motion is achieved if practised daily for 10–15 minutes.

Intensity:

Let the yoga stretches be gradual and gentle. The intensity of a stretch is measured as maximum when a mild discomfort is experienced. Go slow! It leads to injury when muscles are pushed beyond their ability. Let the stretches be constructive, and do not push your body too far. See to it that all major muscle groups are stretched. Concentrate on the body part being stretched and breathe deep long breaths into the focused areas. Never hold the breath while stretching. The breath should be deep, easy and even, and this helps in relaxation. No jerks and no bouncing! Let the stretches be smooth and slow.

Time:

To allow the muscles to lengthen, hold the pose for 10–20 seconds initially. Over a period of time, you can increase the duration to 30 seconds and also increase the number of repetitions. The general goal would be to reach 60 seconds of stretch time per muscle or muscle group. You can also break it up into 1*60/2*30/4*15.

Type:

There are two types: static postures and dynamic postures.

Static postures are the ones in which the position is held for a period of time, counted in breaths, say 15–20 breaths.

Dynamic postures are characterised by moving in and out of posture repeatedly and simultaneously coordinating the movement with breath.

Almost all postures come under the dynamic and static versions. The beginners are advised to start with a dynamic version, i.e., enter into and come out of postures slowly and with total care, repeating them for 2–3 times. This will allow the body to recover from a posture.

As you advance, you can hold the postures for a longer period of time.

Before I end this chapter, let's quickly revise the ten important reasons to work for your flexibility:

1. Reduce muscle and joint pains and unavoidable fatigue.

2. Decrease the risk of injury by correcting excessively tight areas.

3. Improve posture as it loosens muscles around the chest, hamstrings and lower back and strengthens the opposing muscles.

4. Reverse age-related flexibility crisis.

5. Reduces muscular tensions.

6. Prevent muscle soreness after exercise.

7. Massage internal organs, improve circulation, provide relief from arthritis, constipation, flatulence and yes – help remove extra wrinkles and grey hair.

10. A practitioner who cannot do anything beyond these asanas can be treated for many ailments and get much support with these asanas.

11. Promote recovery of injury and regain normal range of motion faster.

Wish you all the luck in saving your spine, shoulders and knees and get the elasticity that you believed only lucky people have!

CHAPTER 2

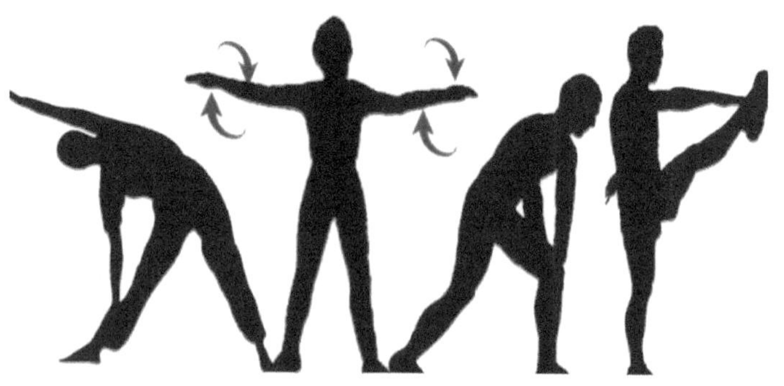

2. LOOSEN UP

To prepare your body for maximum results and minimum injury!

Everyday, to date, I have witnessed yoginis coming 10 minutes late and directly joining our extensive workout. "Warming up is not that important and can be missed", is what they think!

The fact is, you just can't immediately climb on your mat and start your daily practice.

Why?

Because this could lead to injury and, which in turn, can lead to missing your workouts for weeks or even months!

Why so?

Because – working out becomes pretty tough with the following:

1. Pulled hamstrings or groins

2. Tight back or tight hips

3. Stiffness in arms or tight chest muscles

4. Even a pulled face :(

Sorry, the face cannot be pulled, but I had to mention it to establish my point.

What is required is 'warming up'. It is one of the most important things to be done before every workout.

As mentioned earlier, I have always got the vibes from my students that, "it's a mere waste of time to warm up". However, if you do not have time to warm up, then you do not have time to work out.

What happens when you immediately start working out without warming up?

1. The unused muscles, just like the tight rubber bands that are not stretched, get pulled apart very quickly and snap.

2. Stretching cold muscles can pull or injure a joint during the main program of postures.

Benefits of warming up:

1. Warm muscles, tendons and ligaments are more flexible and stretch more easily.

2. Helps blood flow in the muscles involved and consequently prepares you for a full range of motion.

3. Reduces the likelihood of stiffness in the muscles and joints after the session.

Depending upon your goal and fitness level, the warm-up differs. Whatever your goals, the basic goals for every warm-up includes:

1. Warm your joints and all major muscles of the body.

2. Involve conscious breathing so that the mind is centred and remains calm.

3. Include few movements such that the heart rate, breathing and muscle temperature increase slightly.

4. Do a very light static stretching routine at the end of the warm-up (static stretching is gently stretching the muscles and holding them in position for around 20 counts).

Static stretching improves flexibility when compared to injury prevention.

Here is a simple warm-up exercise routine lasting 5 to 7 minutes (with no drama), the flow being in a toe-to-head direction:

Position – Long Sitting

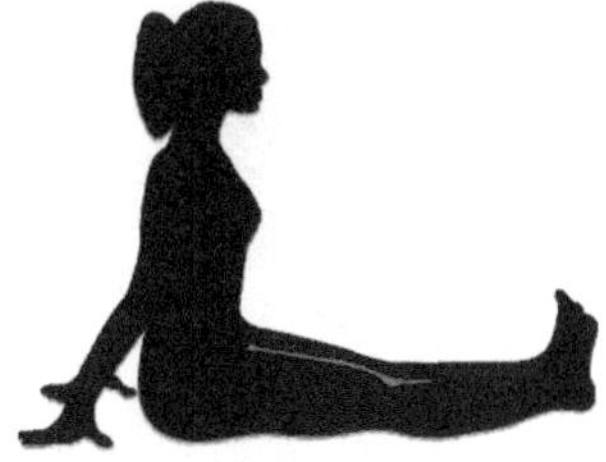

Sit on the floor with your legs stretched out in front, feet together and arms on the mat by the side of the hips.

Stretch the toes, soles and ankles:

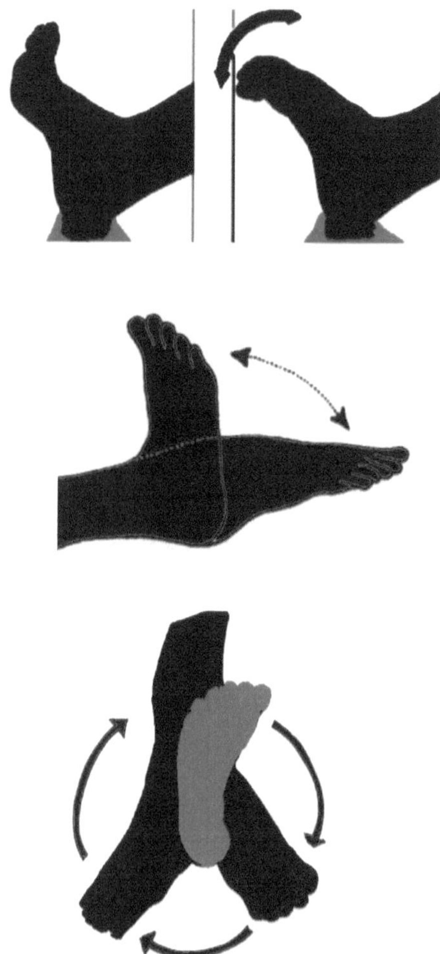

i.   Toes: Keep your feet together, inhale and gently press the toes downwards and exhale and relax the toes and pull them up.

ii. Soles: Keep your feet apart at about 6 to 8 inches, inhale and press the soles forwards slowly. Count 5 and release as you exhale. Now press your soles backwards towards the body. Repeat this for 5 rounds.

iii. Ankle: Rest your feet on the heel and rotate them clockwise and anticlockwise 4-5 times each side.

Knee rotation:

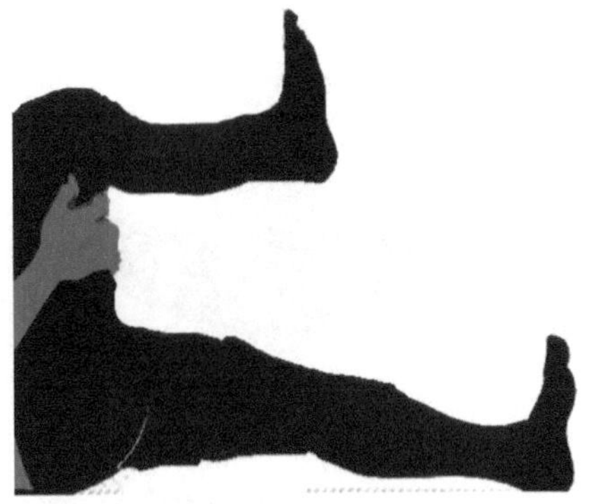

i.   Keep your legs a bit apart.

ii. Fold your right leg, knee facing up, and feet flat on the mat.

iii. Hold your left wrist with your right arm and place it under the right knee.

iv. Raise the right leg up such that the calves are parallel to the mat and knees make 90 degrees angle with the calf of the leg.

v. Rotate the legs clockwise and then anticlockwise 5 to 6 times.

vi. Repeat the same with the other leg.

Thighs, hip muscles and groins – Butterfly stretch:

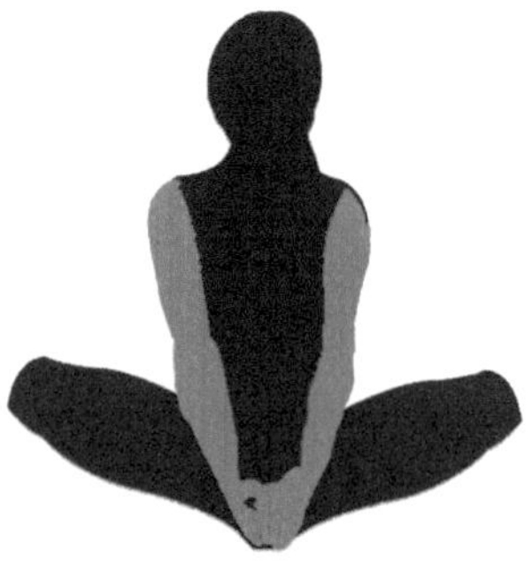

i. Bend the legs from the knees and bring both the soles of your feet together. Interlace fingers and hold the toes. Bring your feet as close as possible to your genitals.

ii. Move the thighs up and down like the wings of a butterfly for around 15 to 20 times.

iii. Hold both the knees with the hands and repeat for 15 times.

iv. Keep pressing your thighs into your groin in this pose instead of pressing the knees down.

Core, thighs, pelvis, psoas, hips, lower back, triceps and biceps –Urdhva Upavista Konasana/Big toe pose:

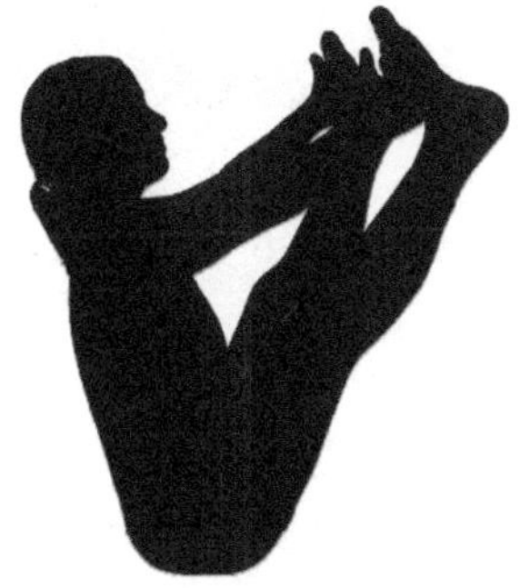

i.   Hook your first two fingers around your big toes.

ii. Exhale and tilt back to remain seated on your sit bones.

iii. Inhale and raise your legs up straight and wide.

iv. Breathe normally.

v.   Gently squeeze your thigh muscles and pull your kneecaps up.

vi. Keep your shoulders beyond the ears, legs active, chest lifted and open and keep lengthening your spine.

Spine stretch:

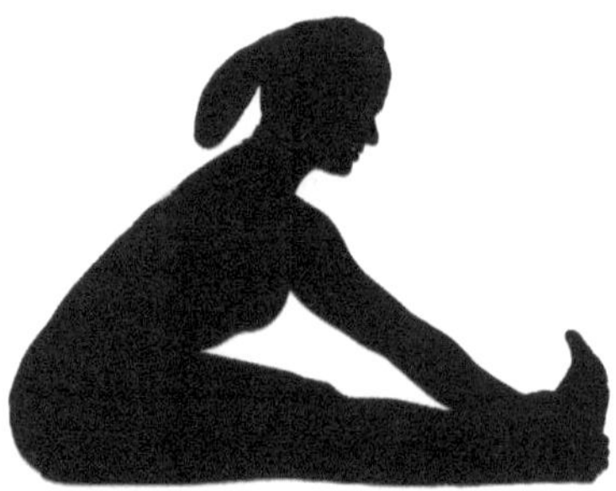

i. Sit in a long position with your arms beside the hips.

ii. Inhale and straighten the spine.

iii. Extend arms in front of you and walk them forward as far as possible to stretch the lower spine.

iv. Exhale and walk your arms backward and sit up tall again in the long sitting position.

v. Repeat the same for 5 to 6 times.vi. Place your arms on either side of the right knee.

vii. Bend forward and walk hands forward to stretch the right side of the spine.

viii. Walk your hands back to sit back in position.

ix. Repeat the same on the left side to stretch the left side of the spine.

x. Sit in a long position.

xi. Place your right hand on the left knee and your left hand behind you.

xii. Inhale and straighten the spine and open the chest.

xiii. Exhale and twist to the left as much as the body permits. The shoulder must remain away from the ears.

xiv. Twist from your navel.

xv. Hold for 3 breaths and repeat on the other side.

Arms, shoulders, hips, quads, core, neck, spine and almost a total body stretch – Chakki Chalanasana/Mill Churning pose:

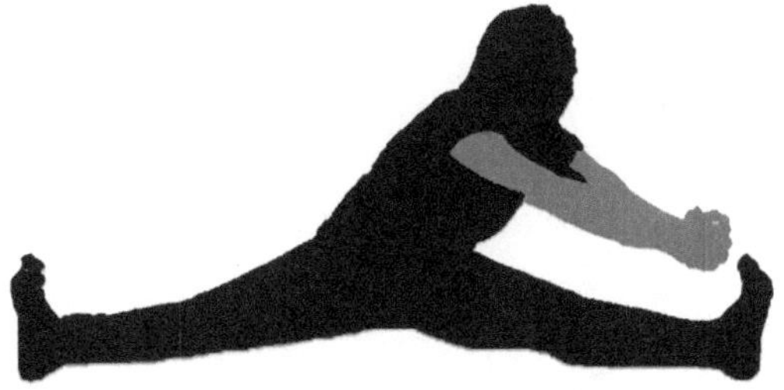

i. Sit on your sit bones with your legs splayed apart.

ii. Clasp your hands and raise them in front of you at shoulder level.

iii. Inhale and bend forward from your hips.

iv. The legs remain silent and the neck remains long in line with the head and shoulders.

v. Rotate your torso from the right to the left, lengthening your spine as you do so.

vi. Look straight and do not look down.

vii. Inhale as you go from right to left and exhale as you go from left to right. Make 8 to 10 rounds clockwise and 8 to 10 rounds anticlockwise.

Position: Standing

Stand in an upright position with shoulders squared and away from your ears (this is done by outward rotation of the shoulders).

Neck exercises:

a. i. Make a fist of your right hand with the thumb in.

ii. Bring the fist under your chin.

iii. Inhale and press your chin upwards and pause for two counts (the fist should not move).

iv. Exhale and press the chin downwards (gently touching the fist) and pause for two counts.

v. Repeat the same 4 to 5 times.

b. i. Keeping the neck long and chin raised, inhale and turn the head towards the right. Pause for one count.

   ii. Exhale and bring it back to the centre.

   iii. Inhale and turn the head towards the left and pause for one count.

   iv. Exhale and bring it back to the centre.

   v. Repeat the same 3 to 4 times on each side.

c. i. Hold your left shoulder with your right palm and pull your chin in.

   ii. The neck should stay long with your head held upright.

   iii. Slowly turn your head towards your left shoulder. The chin shoud now be parallel to the left shoulder.

   iv. Gaze towards your left.

   v. Press the head towards the right shoulder (as if you are trying to pull your right ear towards your right shoulder).

   vi. Gently force your ear towards the shoulder.

   vii. Gaze up and let the neck sit in this position for 5 counts.

viii. The stretch is felt on the neck muscle on the opposite side.

ix. Repeat the same on the other side, with 4 repetitions on each side.

Caution: The exercises above have to be done gently without haste and without any jerks.

Shoulders and arms

Stand with feet slightly apart

Shoulder rotations:

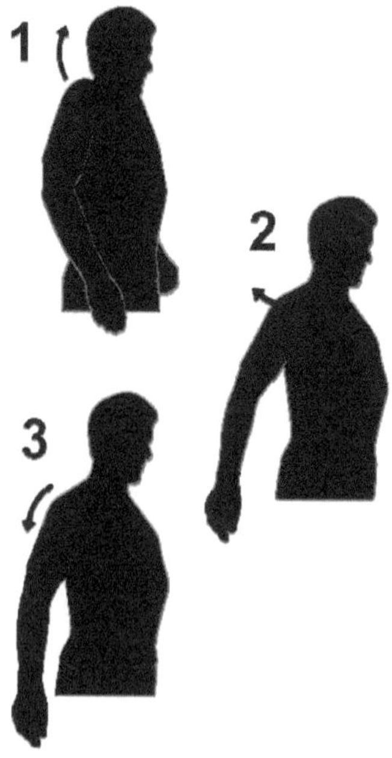

i. Raise your left shoulder to the ear, move it back-
    wards, downwards and around in one continuous
    motion. This completes one round. Repeat the
    move 5 to 6 times and switch directions.

ii. Repeat the same with the other shoulder.

The back, chest, abs and the rest of the body should
remain silent and only the shoulders should move.

a. Arm warmers:

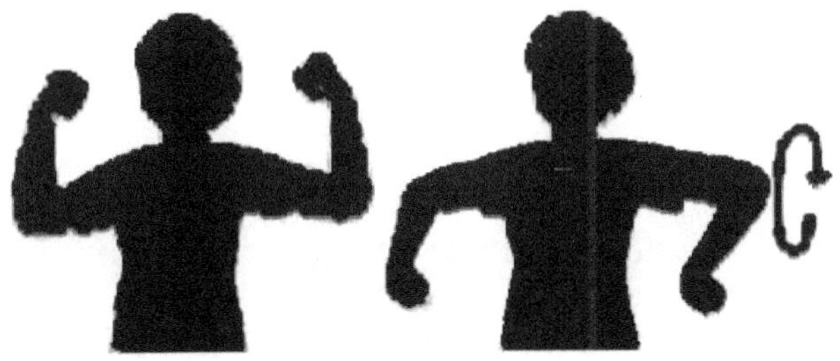

i. Keep your forearms folded towards the shoulders
    and fists closed and facing the biceps.

ii. Exhale, open and stretch your arms (in line with your
    shoulders) with a gentle jerk and simultaneously
    open your fists and stretch your fingers.

iii. Fold your arms again and repeat the same 5 to
    6 times.

b. i. Fold your arms and bring your palms above the chest, palms facing down, with the tips of the middle fingers facing each other.

   ii. Gently open your arms, stretch them and straighten them to your sides in line with the shoulders (palms should remain facing down).

   iii. The arms should make a T with your body.

   iv. Fold them back and bring the palms above the chest and repeat this for 5 to 6 repetitions.

c. i. Stretch out your arms to make a T with your body.

   ii. Make a fist with your thumb in.

   iii. Extend your arms to your sides in line with shoulders.

   iv. Fold your forearm so that it forms a 90-degree angle with the upper arm.

The upper arm should be parallel to the mat.

   v. Fold your forearm down from the elbow, until the front side of your forearm is parallel to the mat.

   vi. Maintain the 90-degree angle between the forearm and the upper arm.

   v. Raise the forearm back to position.

The upper arms, shoulders, neck and other parts of the body should remain silent and only the forearm and fist should move.

Fingers, wrist and forearm:

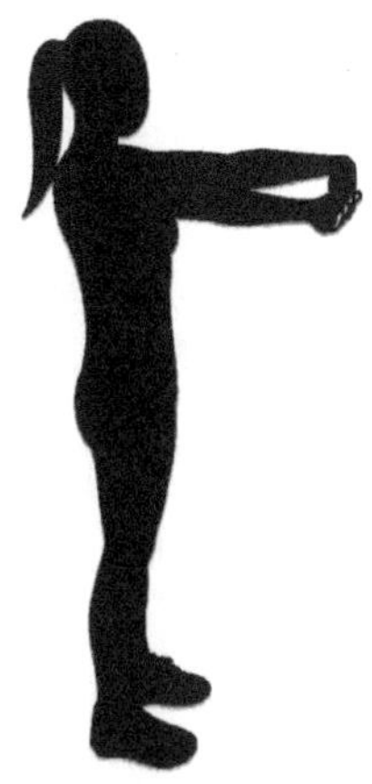

a. i. Keep your right arm in front of you, with your elbow straight and palm facing the roof.

   ii. Stretch all your five fingers.

  iii. Now with the left palm placed on your right palm (making a cross of the palms), gently press all the five fingers of the right palm downwards and backwards, towards your body.

   iv. This pressing should stretch the muscles of the right palm, right wrist and right forearm.

     v.   Hold the position for 10 counts and release the stretch.

    vi.   Repeat the same with the other hand.

b.   i.   Keep your right arm again in front of your body with your elbow straight and palm facing the mat.

    ii.   With the left palm placed on the back of the right palm, making a cross again, gently press the fingers down and towards your body.

   iii.   This stretches the muscles of the right palm, right wrist, and the outer forearm.

    iv.   Hold the position for 10 counts and release the stretch.

     v.   Repeat the same with the other hand.

c.   i.   Keep your hands extended in front of our body and palms facing down.

    ii.   Make a fist with the thumb in.

   iii.   Open the fist and spread the fingers wide and stretch them.

    iv.   Close the fist with the thumb in and keep repeating.

     v.   Repeat the same 5 times.

Torso rotation

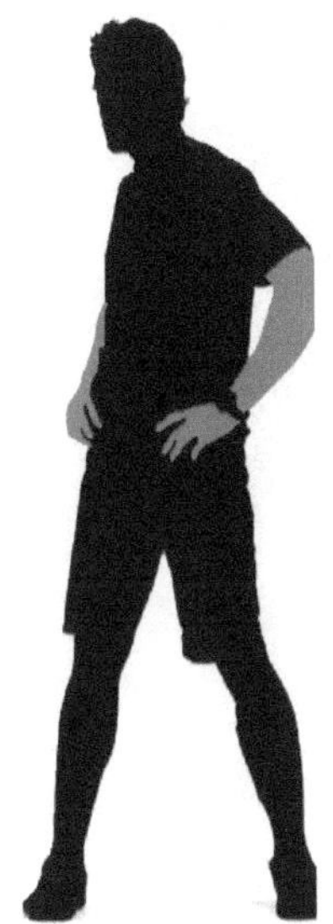

i.   Stay in a standing position, head straight and hands on your hips.

ii. Keep your feet shoulder-width apart and chest lifted up.

iii. Rotate torso at 90 degrees to your right, keeping your hips stable.

iv. Return back and rotate the same way to the left.

v.   Repeat the movements for 10 counts on each side.

Leg swing

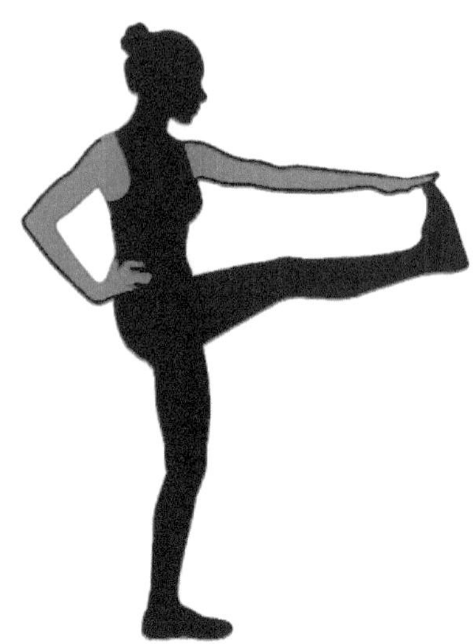

Increases range of motion in the glutes, hip joints, hip flexors, quads, arms and IT bands.

i. Stay in a standing position, with your abs contracted and fully engaged.

ii. Lift up the right leg.

iii. Swing it up straight as far as you can without moving your torso.

iv. Simultaneously extend arms towards the right and reach for the right toes.

v. Bring the leg back down and your arm beside the body.

vi. Swing up again and extend your arm to touch the toes.

vii. Repeat this 10 times and switch legs.

Standing windmill stretch

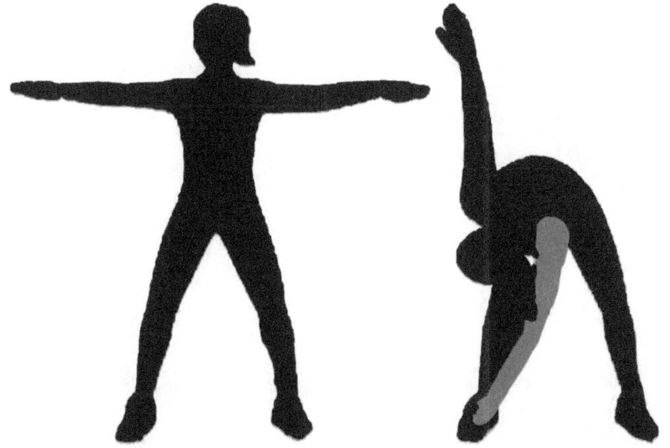

Improves the side-to-side movements and opens up chest and shoulders and facilitates deep breathing.

i. In standing position, widen your legs about twice the shoulder width apart.

ii. Bend from the hips and turn your torso towards your right leg.

iv. Bring your left arm down either flat on the mat

or inside of your right foot and simultaneously lift the right arm as high as possible.

v. Reverse this movement and do it on the left side.

vi. Continue on alternate sides for 10 repetitions on each side.

Caution: Breathe normally when you stretch and do not hold your breath.

Be slow and gentle in your movements.

Face forward and keep your shoulders relaxed.

Stretch as far as you are comfortable.

Finally not to forget, stretch both sides of the body with an equal intensity on each side.

Your warm-up should not fatigue you; therefore listen to your body's cues when you warm up.

Remember this is only one aspect of your workout! Therefore, enjoy your warm-up exercise routine and then get into the child pose until the class begins.

As important as the warming up is before each workout, so is the cooling down after each workout.

Don't forget to <u>cool down</u> at the end of each session.

Meet you in the next chapter to understand a cooling exercise regime.

CHAPTER 3

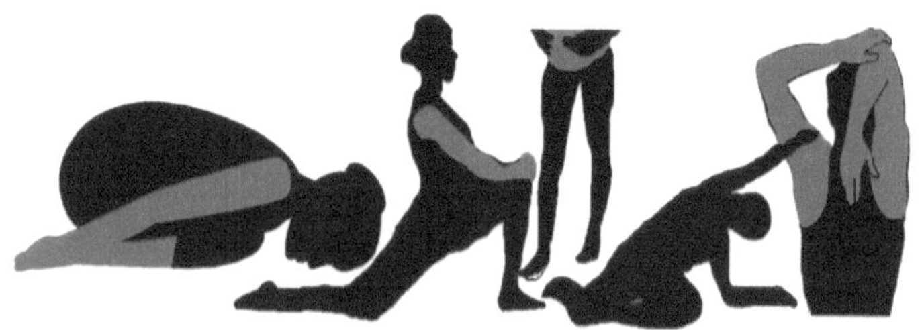

3. COOL DOWN

Unwinding post-workout is as important as warming up pre-workout!

My smart and busy yoginis often try to cut down the workout time by skipping the cooling down. They have a list of reasons to escape the final 5 to 7 minutes of cooling down and miss the fact that a cool-down session can make or break a good workout regime, just like a good warm-up would.

WHY?

Simply because, when we stop suddenly after an intensive workout, the fast pumping heart has to stop suddenly. This means that there can be a sudden drop in blood pressure. Also, this pools blood in the expanded blood vessels of your legs and feet. There are high chances of you feeling dizzy, fainting, or even 'passing out' (depending upon the intensity of your workout).

As warm-ups prepare our body for strenuous workouts, cooling down aids the sore muscles, joints and the body to bounce back to normal.

Cooling down has the following benefits:

- Slows the heart rate and stretches warm muscles.

- Prevents muscle tightness and alleviates muscle soreness.

- Relaxes the mind and physiological systems of the body.

- Power yoga sessions followed by a long and good cool-down sequence helps to flush out the lactic acid, which otherwise is a cause for muscle pain and swelling.

A fine cooling-down session broadly requires the following:

- Light static stretching sequence of asanas that lowers the pulse.

- Focussing attention on the breath during the asana practice to help oxygenate the system.

- Holding each stretch for 10–20 counts or more.

Triceps and shoulder stretch

a. Overhead triceps stretch

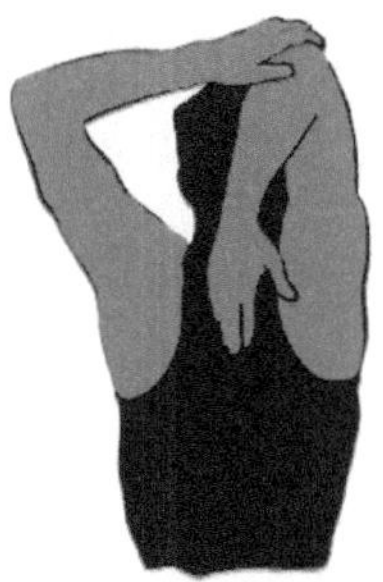

a. Raise your right arm straight up to the roof and bend at the elbow to bring the palm towards the centre of your shoulders, and rest the fingers along the spine.

b. With your left arm, hold your right elbow and push it towards the centre and downwards

c. Hold for 10 counts and repeat on the other side

d. You can do this either standing or sitting.

b. Horizontal stretch

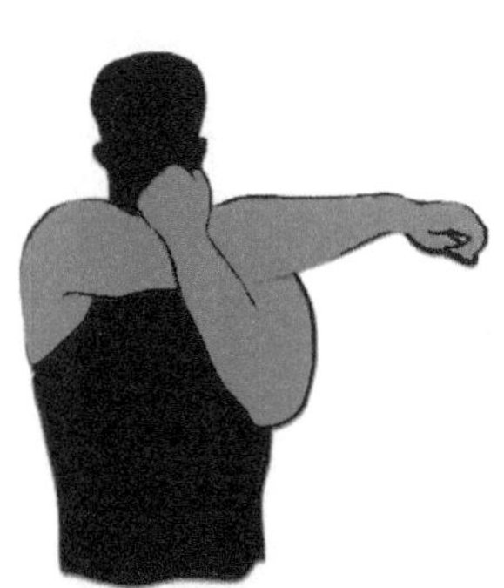

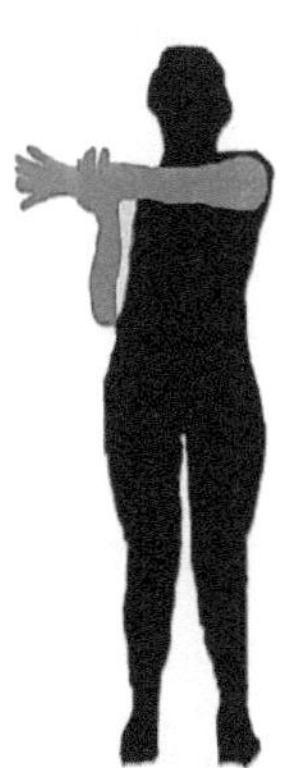

a. Extend the right hand forward and straight, perpendicular to the body.

b. Gently bring it across the body.

c. Extend the left arm diagonal to the body and lock the right arm at the right elbow by folding the left arm 90° at the elbow.

d. Press the right arm into the chest and over the left.

e. Hold for 10 counts.

Side mermaid

Obliques, arms, shoulders and torso:

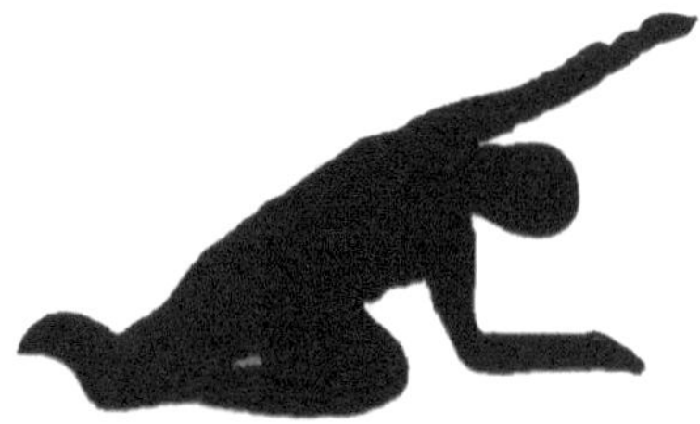

a. Sit on your right side, bending your knees in such a way that the right sole touches the inner thighs of the left leg.

b. Bend onto the right side and place the right forearm a little away from your right waist, with fingers of the arm pointing forward.

c. Reach the left arm overhead and extend it straight such that the fingers, the arms and the left side are all in one line. Keep the arm close to the ears.

d. Stay in the pose for 5 counts.

e. Rise up gently and now bend on the left side and hold your left ankle with your left arm and reach the right arm overhead. Keep the arm close to the ears.

f. See to it that the hips stay anchored onto the ground when you bend on both sides.

g. Repeat 5 times on both sides.

Knee squeezes

Upper, middle and lower back muscles:

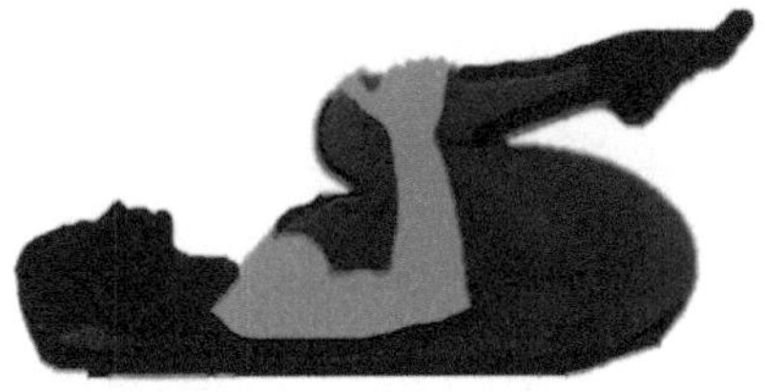

a. Lie on your back.

b. Bend both your knees and hold them with your arms.

c. Gently press the knees and bring them towards your chest.

d. Relax your neck and shoulders.

e. Hold the pose for 10 to 15 counts.

Calf stretch

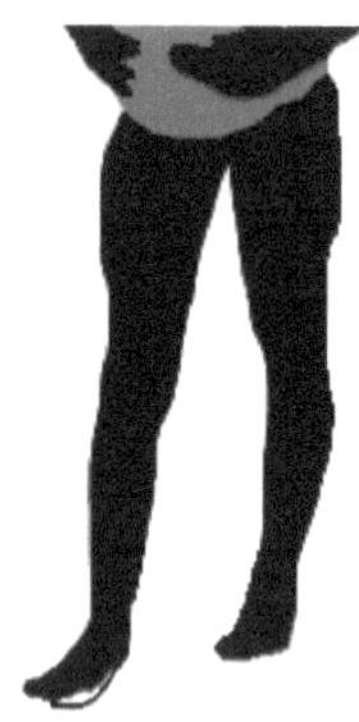

a. Stand with your feet a little apart and one behind the other.

b. The knee behind should be slightly bent and the other leg should be straight out in front.

c. Lean forward.

d. Simultaneously raise the toes of the leg in front and point them towards your body.

e. Hold your waist with your arms.

f. Keep your back straight.

g. Stay in position for 10 to 15 counts.

h. Repeat by swapping the legs.

Lizard pose

Hip flexors, quads and hamstrings:

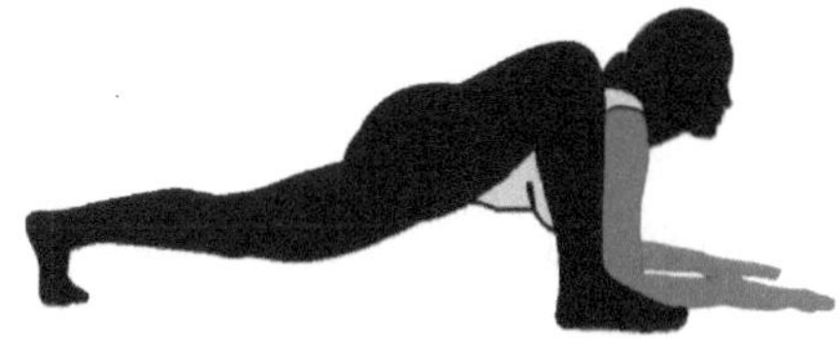

a. Begin in a low lunge with your right leg forward and left leg behind.

b. Rest the left knee down (modified) or you can keep it off the mat (challenging), and keep the right knee stacked over the right ankle.

c. If the knee is off the mat, then the toes should stay rooted on the mat.

d. Bring the right hand inside of the right foot, and keep both the palms close to each other near the inside of the right foot.

e. Bring the front foot out a bit wider.

f. For it to be more challenging, you can place the forearms down.

g. Lengthen the spine and keep it as long as you can.

h. The shoulders should remain levelled.

i. Sink the chest down, open your chest and gaze forward.

j. Remain in the pose for 20 to 30 seconds.

k. Swap legs.

Happy baby pose

Inner thighs, hips, groins, ankles and entire spine, especially the sacral region:

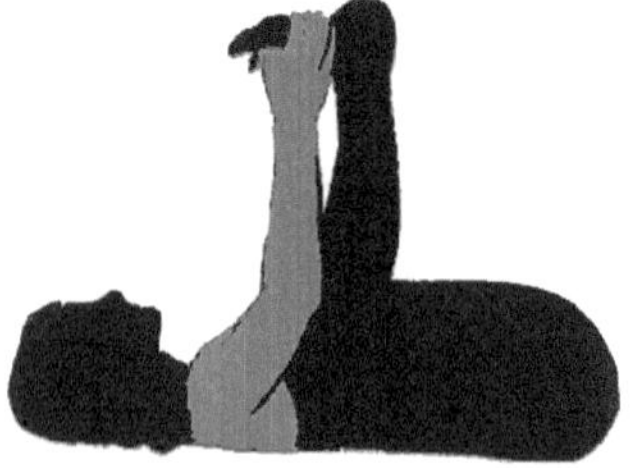

a. Lie in a supine position.

b. Bring both knees to the chest and raise the lower legs upwards such that the soles face the roof.

c. Bringing your arms from the outside of your knees, hold the soles with your respective arms.

d. The head should remain on the mat.

e. Tucking your chin slightly into the chest, press your bent legs down.

f. The shoulders, the back of the neck and spine should be flat and pressed down onto the mat.

g. For a deeper stretch in the hip, let the legs open a little wider.

Quadriceps stretch

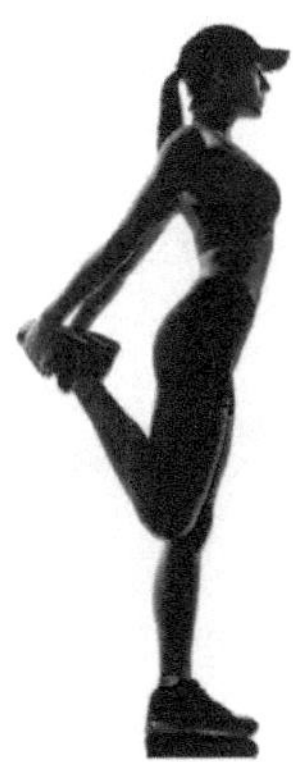

a. Begin in tadasana.

b. Bend your right leg backward and bring the right heel towards your hips.

c. Hold onto the right ankle with either both hands or just the right hand. You can even take the support of the wall or chair.

d. Pull in your abdominal muscles and stand straight.

e. See that the knees are kept close to each other.

f. Keep your shoulders relaxed and open the chest.

g. Stay in the pose for 20 counts.

h. To come out of the pose release, the right leg and repeat with the other leg.

Wide-legged child pose

Relieves back and neck strain, relieves stress and fatigue and calms the brain.

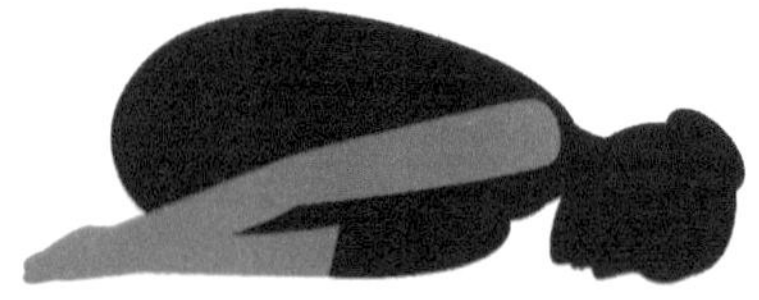

a. Sit in between the heels, spreading the knees wide and big toes touching each other.

b. Sit up straight, lengthening your spine up.

c. Slowly bend down from your hips, keeping your torso straight.

d. The neck and spine should remain long as you bow down.

e. Extend your arms in the front, spreading your fingers wide and your palms facing downwards.

f.   Rest the forehead gently on the mat.

g.   Soften your lower back, broaden the upper back and ease away all the tension from your neck, shoulders and arms.

h.   You can either close your eyes or gaze down and inward.

i.   Stay in the pose for 20 counts.

j.   To come out of the pose, slowly walk your arms back and walk your torso back and make it upright.

Your body is transiting from working hard to resting. Therefore, remember to stretch only till you feel a slight pull and not feel pain.

Breathe mindfully and take deep breaths, as your body needs oxygen to relax the tired muscles.

Cooling down your body is the right way to treat your body after a tough workout. Hence, treat it the right way, and it will thank you forever!

CHAPTER 4

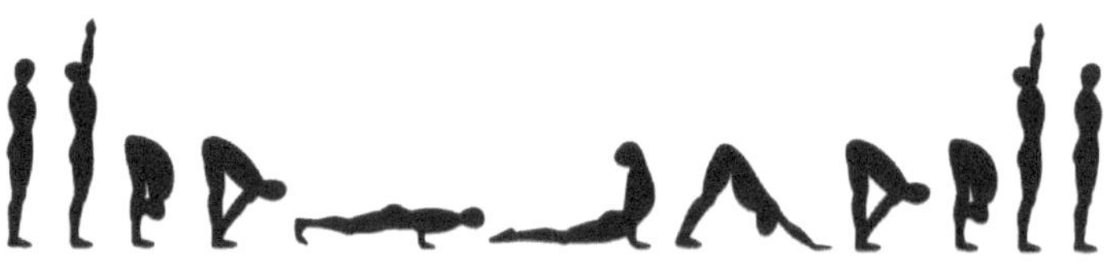

4. FITNESS FOR THE BUSY BEES

We welcome you to the world of surya namaskars.

"So caught up with my busy schedule that I can't spare one whole hour for my workout!'

This is what the so-called busy bees say, but is it not that anyone can find some spare time unless they work 16 hours – 7 days a week? (IT people, do you?) Maybe they have additional commitments such as family and other social responsibilities. Whatever the reason may be, if you can take out a bare minimum of 20 minutes from your daily schedule, THEN READ ON.

One famous vinyasa that particularly hogs the limelight when it comes to multiple benefits in limited workout time is 'surya namaskars.' It not only helps in sculpting your body and getting into an envious frame, but also helps in gaining overall flexibility and stamina, getting flatter abs, stronger spine and firmer muscles, promotes postural re-integration, endorses cardiovascular health and detoxifies the organs (need I say more?).

Whether it is Kareena Kapoor's size zero avatar or Shilpa Shetty's seductive curves or the fit and exemplary bodies of divas such as Jennifer Aniston, Lady Gaga or Demi

Moore, they are all the results of religiously following the practice of Surya Namaskar.

This dynamic yogic posture sequence is a series of 12 physical postures that prove to be a thorough balance of strengthening and stretching postures. It can be done in 3 paces:

1. Slow for flexibility,

2. Medium for toning of muscles, and

3. Fast as a cardio workout.

The practice involves the following:

- Stretching upwards and downwards

- Stretching forwards and backwards

- Carrying your entire weight sequentially on your lower body and then on your upper body.

Every pose is followed by a counter-pose.

Now, this opposed principle of biomechanics creates a contraction and release of opposing muscles that produces levers and loads, which tones, stretches and strengthens the muscles of the entire body and increases circulation in them.

Surya namaskar is in itself a complete form of yoga (like other forms) and ends up working on all the five different aspects such as flexibility, strength, cardiovascular endurance, body composition and weight. The best thing about the practice of surya namaskars is that it can be done by anyone, as the postures can be customized based on body type, medical histories, breathing habits and levels of strength and flexibility. For people who are 'busy bees' and who always face a time crunch, it is an established boon! When you practise sun salutations slowly, it helps in gaining flexibility and is relaxing and meditative. When practised at a fast pace, it turns out to be a good cardiovascular workout and aids to quick weight loss.

One round of sun salutation consists of 12 yoga poses. One set consists of two rounds of sun salutation: first stepping backwards with your right leg, and in the next round you step backwards with the left foot, making an alternating leg sequence. If one practises two rounds of surya namaskar every day, it will mean that the body has gone through 730 rounds of surya namaskar a year, which I believe is enough to influence the musculoskeletal structure of the body. Furthermore, when you do 12 sets of sun salutation, you are completing 12 sets x 2 rounds, i.e., 24 rounds. Each round comprises of 12 yoga poses, which translates to 288 yoga poses and that too within 10–12 minutes. Isn't it amazing to complete 288 powerful yoga postures in a span of just 10–12 minutes?

Now coming to the calories, one set of surya namaskar burns approximately 13.90 calories for a person of average weight.

The general calorie burn out in 30 minutes of weight lifting workout is 199 calories,

a game of Basketball is 265 calories.

a game of football is 298 calories

best cardio workouts, such as cycling, is 331 calories

rock climbing is 363 calories

and running (7.5mph) is 414 calories

Bingo! Just 15 minutes of Surya namaskars (minimum one set in one minute) burns around 210 calories. This with a bonus of completing more than 288 powerful yoga postures in the same time. Isn't it amazing!

Not forgetting the fact that it can be customized according to body type, this amazing vinyasa can be practised by anyone for shedding the extra flab.

However, is surya namaskara just a number or mere physical exercises for burning calories? No, it's far more than that because each posture of the sequence offers its own set of benefits, and when each asana blends into a sequence harmoniously, the overall benefits exceed the sum of its parts!

Summarizing the overall benefits of this proven vitalizing sequence:

- It stimulates and assists the vital organs such as the heart, liver, intestine, stomach, chest, throat and legs.

- It boosts respiratory capacity, improves cardio-vascular functioning and stimulates the digestive system.

- It promotes strength, vitality, lightness and agility.

- It gives relief from mental strain, stress and emotional anxiety.

- It improves muscle flexibility.

- It reverses osteoporosis, secretes synovial fluids in the synovial tissues that lubricate the joints, maintains the cartilage and removes debris of the joints.

- Prevents loss of hair and greying.

- Tones up the nervous system and improves memory.

- The one exercise that works directly on our glands, optimizes metabolism, aids in pain-free menstrual periods and regulates healthy levels of vitamin D.

- Acts as a detoxifying agent, by getting rid of an enormous quantity of carbon dioxide and other toxic gases.

- With the regular practice of surya namaskar and meditation, the solar plexus, which is known as the second brain, increases from the size of an almond to the size of a palm. This expansion develops our sixth sense and makes us more clear and focussed.

As darkness cannot last in the presence of light, illness cannot prevail in the presence of a regular practice of sun salutations.

After several rounds, it also helps in clearing the clogs in the nostrils, and breath flows evenly through them. This aids a healthy pattern of left and right nostril dominance to alternate during the day.

To sum up, this is a holistic practice for physical, mental and spiritual well-being.

Now the practice:

Namaskarasana (prayer pose)

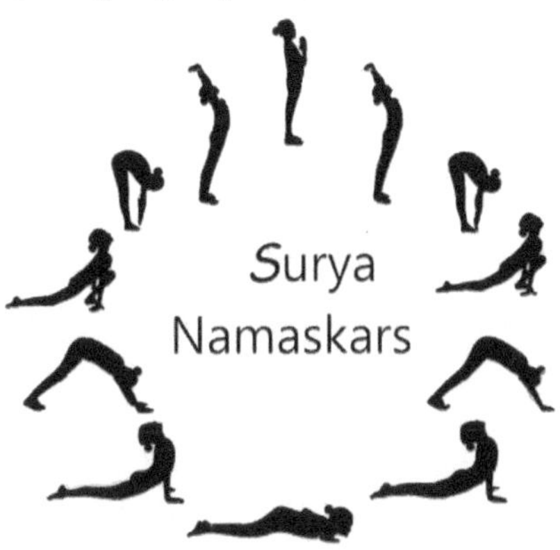

Begin in tadasana (stand about one foot away from the top of the mat).

Bring your palms together in a prayer position in the middle of your chest where your heart is located. Let the breathing be normal and stabilized.

Hastottanasana (raised arms pose)

Extend your arms forward and then above your head.

When your arms reach your ears, breathe in and arch back from your waist.

Push your hips out and let your legs remain straight.

Do not bend your arms from your elbows.

Keep inhaling as you bend back.

Bend back as far as you can.

Remember to bend your head along with your arms once they reach your ears.

Uttanasana (forward bending)

Breathe out, lift up your body, bring your arms back near your ears, and then bend your torso forward from your hips, keeping your hips in line with your heels.

As you bend, engage your core, elongate your neck in line with your spine and bring your chest to your thighs.

The crown of the head is facing the mat

Keep bending down, and if possible, reach down on the mat and place your palms on both sides of your feet.

Try and touch your forehead with your knees.

Beginners can micro-bend their knees. They can also cup their fingers and place the tips on the mat if their palms cannot reach the mat.

You can also reach for your ankles or your shin.

Ashwa sanchalanasana(lunge/equestrian pose)

Breathe in, lower your hips and move your right leg away from your body in a wide backward stretch.

Let your right knee touch the mat.

The toes of your right foot should touch the mat and your heels should face the roof.

Your left leg should be bent at your knees and your left foot should be flat on the mat.

Your left foot should be in between your two palms.

Slightly press your left thigh forward and bring it close to your chest.

Look up and arch back by lifting your chin up.

Dandasana (plank pose)

Hold your breath, bring your left leg back and put it alongside your right leg.

Your knees should remain straight, up and off the mat.

Your spine also should remain straight.

Your whole body should be in one line and parallel to the mat.

Divide the weight of your body equally onto your toes and palms.

Gaze at the mat with your neck remaining long.

Ashtangasana (eight limbs)

Breathe out and gently bring down your knees, chest, chin and forehead on the mat.

Keep your hips slightly off the mat.

Curl your toes inwards.

Your arms should remain close to your body and beside your body.

Your elbows should be parallel to each other and point upwards.

Your palms should be a little under your chest.

Gaze straight.

Bhujangasana (cobra pose)

Breathe in and bring your hips down on the mat.

Lie on your abdomen and bring your palms beside your armpits.

Pressing your hips on the mat, gently raise your chest up.

Press your shoulders down and back, and arch your spine evenly.

Bend backwards as much as you can and gaze up.

Your hips have to remain planted onto the mat and your navel off the mat.

Adho mukha svanasana (downward dog pose)

Exhaling and gently pressing your palms and toes,

raise your knees, back, hips and chest into an inverted 'V' shape.

Relax your head between your arms.

Push your torso and head in and look inwards towards your knees.

Try and touch the heels of your feet on the mat.

The following asanas 9, 10, 11 and 12 are repetitions of asanas 4, 3, 2, and 1.

Ashwa sanchalanasana

(lunge/equestrian pose)

Uttanasana (forward bending)

Hastottanasana (raised arms pose)

Namaskarasana (prayer pose)

This constitutes one round of surya namaskar. One set of surya namaskar consists of two rounds – one leading with the right leg (as in posture 4) and the second leading with the left leg.

The right technique of practising these '12 postures – energizing sequence' involves three important elements:

Right alignment

Flow

Breath connect

Right alignment

It is nothing but positioning your body in an accurate way so that

a. You engage the postural muscles and prevent recruiting other muscles,

b. You prevent pain, discomfort and injury,

c. You reap the comprehensive benefits of the yoga pose.

The flow

Flow is everything that happens between the asanas – the transition from one asana to the other, and that which connects the asanas. The movement from one pose to another is a pose itself and therefore is as important as the pose. The transitions act like seams that connect the pieces of our practice and smoothly complete the practice.

It is said that the practice of surya namaskar is in a waveform, and if you want to flow like a peaceful wave and glide seamlessly from one pose to the other, then here are a few tips:

Focus on the next pose, but do not ignore moments in between the poses.

Let the transitions be mindful, and notice what is happening to your body, mind and breath.

a. When you bend backward in the 2nd pose, see that the head remains positioned in between the arms and does not bend towards the back earlier. Same applies when bending forward in the 3rd pose.

b. When getting into a lunge position, initiate the movement from your leg and feet. Consciously keep stretching your leg by energizing the muscles of your leg. Keep your front knee centred over your ankle.

c. From 4th to 5th – initiate moment from your leg and feet and instead of a knee -jerk let it be a knee-swing reaction

d. Getting into the 6th pose requires gently placing your knees, stomach, chest and chin sequentially down (and keep your hips raised).

e. As you move up into bhujangasana, initiate the transition by changing the position of your feet, so that the movement surges through your leg into your spine. Remember to use your arms to move your rib cage away from your legs and place them in a position that would allow them to remain perpendicular to the floor. Your legs need a continuous spiralling inwards for the full lift of your upper chest.

f. The poses 5, 6, 7 and 8 is a perfect diagonal flow and is like an aircraft that comes down and, instead of landing, rises up.

g. Therefore, from dandasana, which is the 5th pose, we have to rise to downward dog pose, which is the 6th pose. This transition has two options: one is you can initiate the movement by contracting your abdominal muscles, support your spine and move your head first. The second option is to pull your navel into your spine, support your spine and initiate movement from the top of your thighs.

h. The transition to the lunge pose is supposed to be the most difficult, as getting your foot in between your hands requires technique, in addition to strength and flexibility. Few tips for this are

I. Shift your weight from your pelvis to your front leg and lean slightly to one side to bring your foot between your hands.

II. If this is not possible, then take your leg a little back energizing your thigh muscles and your foot, and with a little force bring your foot forward.

III. If your foot stops at a shorter distance, you can just hold your shin and bring your foot forward.

i. To walk forward into uttanasana, initiate the movement by shifting the weight from your pelvis to your front foot. Ground your feet and lift your sit bones as you transit to this pose.

j. To move to the 2nd pose, initiate the transition from the movement of your legs. Relax your neck and strongly focus on the grounding of your legs, the lengthening of the spine, the extension of the arms, and the balance between the elongation of your right and left waists.

k. To return back to the start bring your attention to centering your body from the front of your heels to the crown of your head.

l. Keep your core engaged throughout.

Experiment with the above suggestions and discover what works best for you, because, all in all, transitions in yoga are as hard as they are in life!

Do not rush through the transitions, because if you have poor alignment in a transition and if you move quickly through it again and again, then you risk injury.

When you happen to pick up the pace, avoid jerk in any pose. Let the movements be fluid and graceful.

Lastly, accept your physical limitations, and do not force to the point of strain.

Breath connect

As with alignment and transition, the breath is also a critical component in the practice of surya namaskar. When movements are coordinated with breath it aids the following:

- Connecting the body and the mind
- Controlling movements and reducing chances of injury
- Eliminates joint compression from one's posture and endows muscular strength
- Seamless flow in movement through the practice.

How and when to use breath in the practice?

As there is a natural tendency for the chest and abdomen to expand on inhalation and contract on exhalation, when you bend forward, exhale, and when lifting or opening your chest, inhale

When does breath take place?

It takes place during transitions. Yes, not during the asana, but in between the asanas.

Then what do you do in the asanas? Do whatever you want but never hold your breath.

Breathe normally and not in ujjayi. Be aware of each exhale and inhale, and let it be synchronized, slow, smooth and effortless.

Breathe slowly, gently and effortlessly. Let the breath be in harmony with each body movement.

Word of caution: As we have varied lifestyles, medical histories, health conditions, breathing habits and levels of strength and flexibility, it is always advised to practise under a yoga instructor, wherein she/he shall analyze the personal medical history and health conditions and therein customize the practice accordingly.

CHAPTER 5

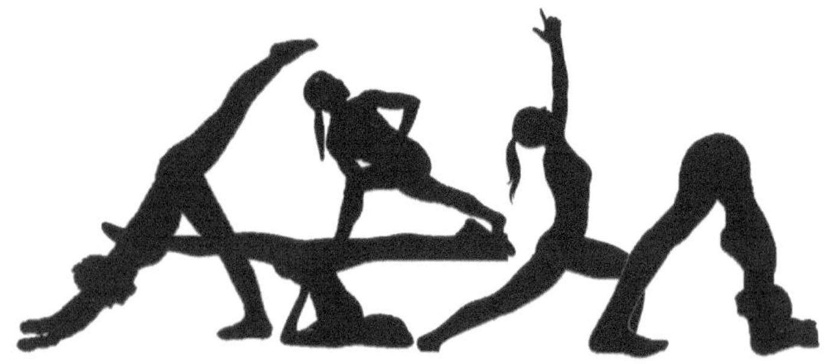

5. CARDIO YOGA

I want something that can give me a good sweat and torch my heart beat high!

I love yoga but I love cardio too!

I have no time (and patience) for one hour of yoga or other workouts!

If any of the above is YOU then I suggest, you try Cardio Yoga. This workout is a flow that combines the benefits of cardio with the strengthening, sculpting, stretching benefits of yoga and what makes it fun is, it has active repetitions - all these together coalesce into an effective workout which is about 20 to 30 minutes (good for people who always crib with lack of time) and if you have time, then you can repeat the sequence twice or thrice according to your convenience

Cardio yoga is a form of circuit training wherein you involve both the upper and lower body, and the exercises are dynamic and quick. They tone muscles all over the body and prove to be a well-rounded exercise program that ends up burning higher calories and fat in a short amount of time, and at the same time increases strength and bone density. When yoga practice is properly integrated with cardio - you get the best of both worlds!

You end up losing 250 to 500 calories (based on experience), and the conditions applied for this are:

- How hard you work?
- How much you weigh?
- The time factor?

Essentially it is an exercise program that combines :

- Fat burning benefits of **HIIT**
- Pumping up the heartbeat, raising metabolism, higher calorie burn and fat burn with **Cardio**
- Toning, sculpting and stretching benefits of **Power Yoga**
- It's a bodyweight workout and therefore can be done anywhere

Thus without getting into more details of How / Why this combination of exercise program works, let's get ready to pump the blood up, torch the heartbeat hard, sweat and burn calories.

The workouts are of 20 and 30 minutes

The 20-minutes workout:

- If you want to squeeze it in between your lunch break in the office or

- If you could set your morning alarm 20 minutes early

The 30 minutes is, if you want a metabolic raise and sculpt, tone and stretch while the dinner is getting ready

Before starting the main workout, it's necessary to do a few dynamic warm-up exercises. Dynamic exercises are movements that get our body moving to help our joints and muscles go through a full range of motion.

These are the 7 quick dynamic warm-up exercises to help you improve your workout performance and reap the workout rewards

They should not take more than 5 minutes.

Arm Circles

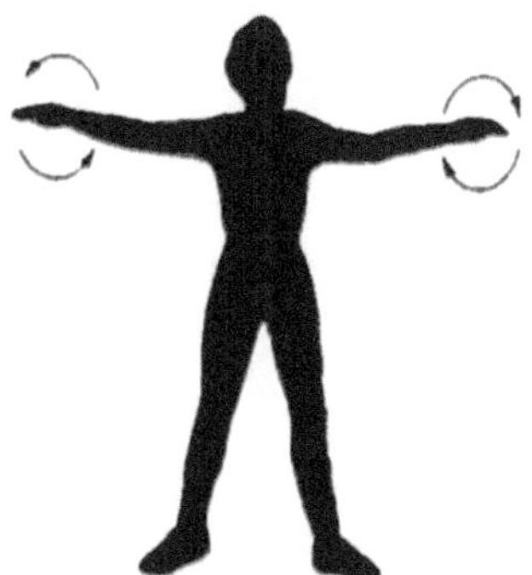

1. Stand with feet hip-distance apart

2. Extend arms sideways in line with your shoulders

3. Circle your arms in clockwise directions, start with smaller circles for 3 rounds and the next 3 rounds work up to larger ones. Reverse directions to anticlockwise similarly

Walking Jacks

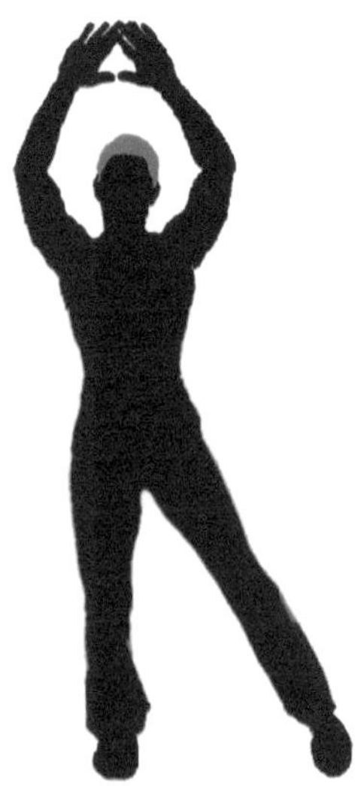

1. Stand with feet together

2. Step one leg out to the sides

3. Simultaneously raise arms up overhead to opposite diagonals

4. Balance body weight equally on both the feet

5. Step in and repeat the same with the other legs

6. Total counts of 20 on each side

Standing Toe Touch

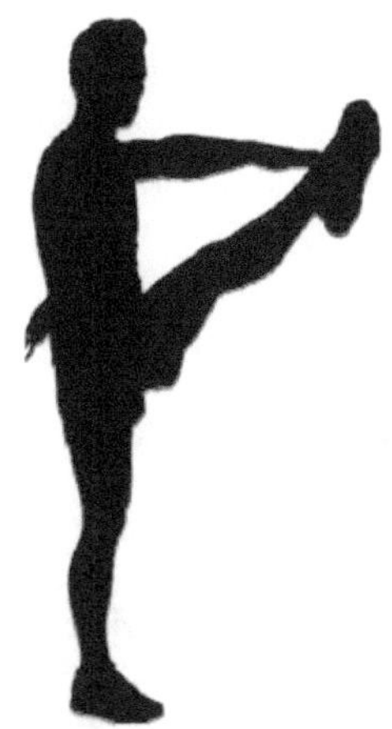

1. Stand with feet hip-distance apart

2. Swing your right leg forward and up

3. Simultaneously extend left arm to touch your right toes

4. Swing the left leg forward and up

5. Simultaneously extend right arm to touch your left toes

6. Repeat for 10 counts with each leg

Hip Rotations

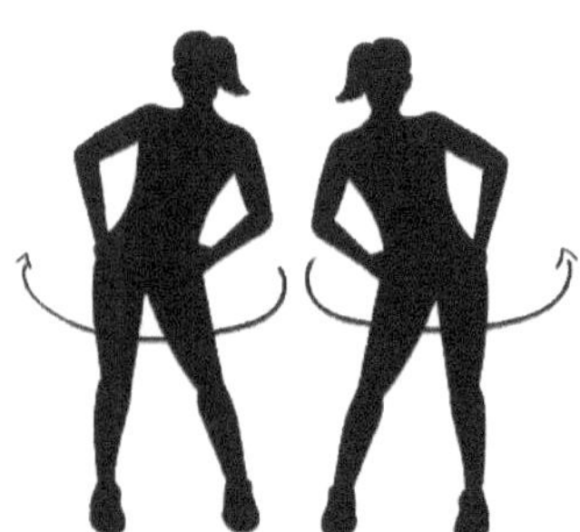

1. Stand with feet wider than your shoulder-width distance

2. Place your hands on the hip

3. Open your chest and shoulders away from the ears (external rotation of shoulders)

4. Move hips to your right (clockwise) make a circle and move from side to back and then to the left side and finally to the front

5. This completes one rotation

6. 8 rotations in a similar way

7. Move hips to your right side (anticlockwise), make a circle and move from side to the front and then to the left side and finally to the back

8. This completes one rotation

9. 8 rotations in a similar way

Body Weight Squats

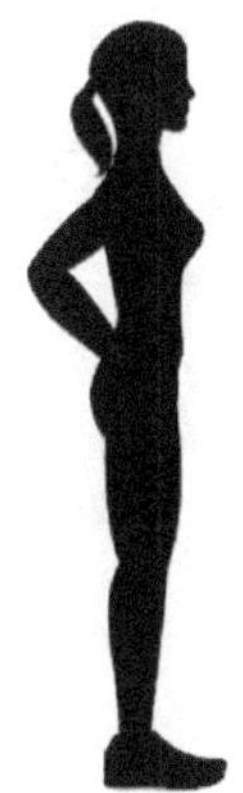 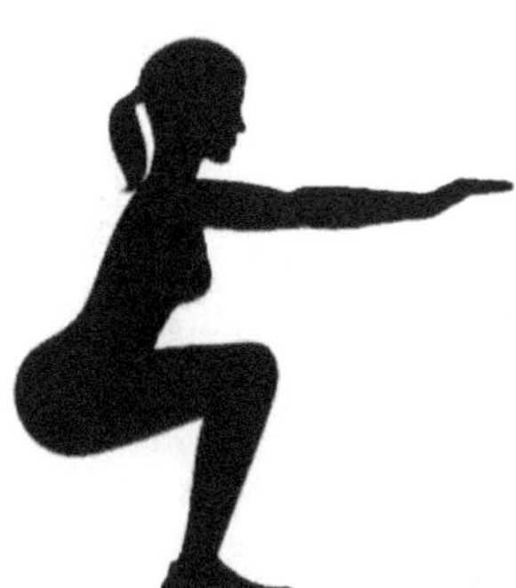

1. Stand with feet wider than hip-width (the distance between the hips) apart

2. Point your toes slightly outwards

3. Engaging your core, push your hips down by putting effort on your thighs and keeping your knees soft

4. Push them down till the thighs are almost parallel to the mat

5. The torso can flex forward slightly

6. Keep engaging the core and keep spine straight flat

7. Press the midfoot and straighten legs to stand up

8. Do 20 to 25 repetitions

Walk Down Planks

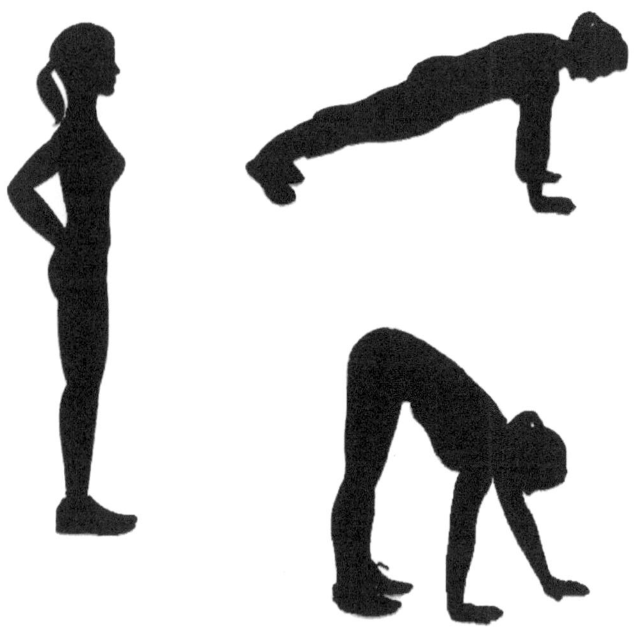

1. Stand in tadasana

2. Push hips down, bend knees gently and place your palms down on the mat

3. Walk them out until you are in a plank position

4. Now walk your arms back up to a standing position

5. This is one round

6. Complete 8 rounds of the walk down planks

Skater Jumps

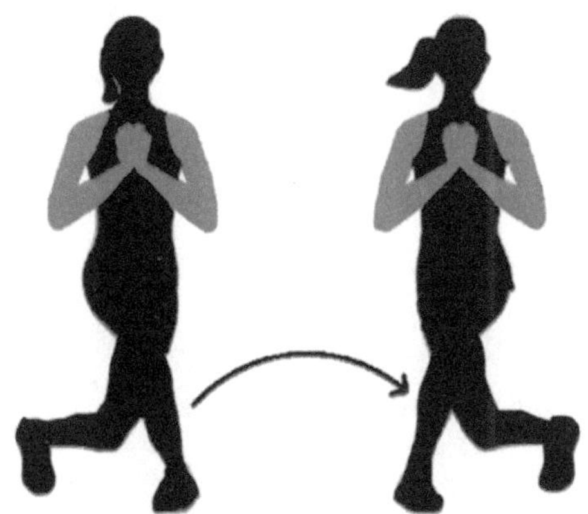

1. Stand with legs hip-width distance

2. Hop to your right and land on your right foot

3. The right leg is bent at the knee at approx 90* or more

4. Sweep the left foot diagonally behind the right leg

5. You can either place the left leg down on its toes or keep it flying, bend the legs at the knees (the shin is parallel to the mat in this position)

6. Interlace fingers of the arms and place them in the middle of the chest

7. Hop now to the left side and land on your left toes.

8. 10 repetitions on both sides

Make it a habit to do these warm-up exercises before you start your main workout routine. These exercises will act as part of your main workout as you will be doing the same functional movements in your main workout. These seven warm-up moves will keep you injury-free and will keep you mobile and supple

Let's get started with our cardio yoga workout which shall help you burn more calories and more fat in less time!

Module 1

Chair Pose To Chair Twist Pose

Chair Pose

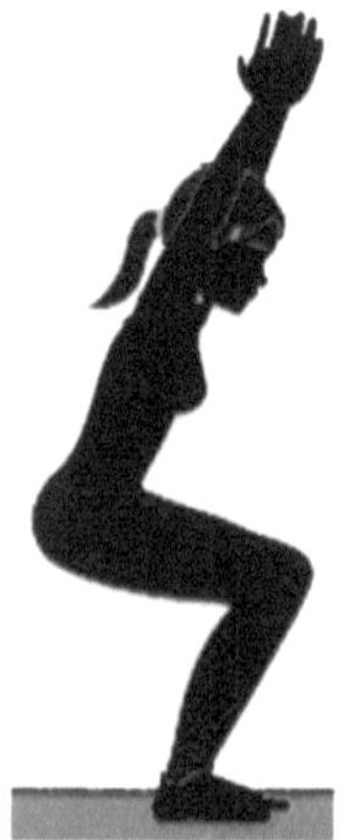

TO

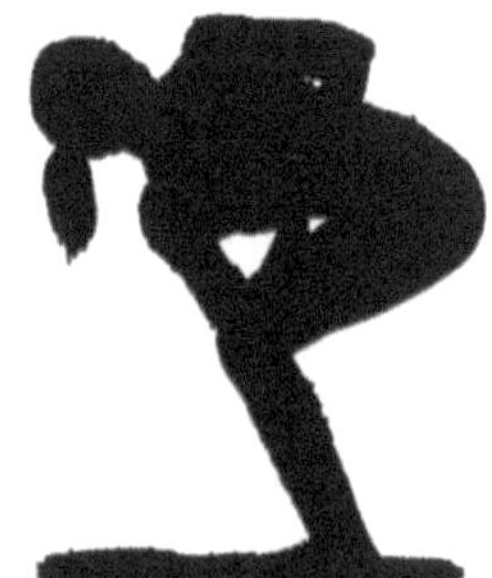

1. Begin in tadasana

2. From tadasana, gently extend both arms forward, elbows facing to the sides and palms facing each other

3. Slowly fold your knees, first to a smaller degree and then deepening, push your hips down gently until your buttocks are in line with the folded knee line

4. As you fold knees and push hips down, gently raise your arms straight up in line with the ears

5. Keep drawing inner thighs down and back, and engage your quads (upper thigh)

6. Also, engage the calves and ankles

7. Feet is hip-width distance and push weight into heels

8. Imagine you are sitting on an invisible chair

9. Gaze forward or up at the thumb

10. Stay in the pose for 2 counts

11. Get into the twisted chair pose

Keep lengthening your spine and that will help you balance

Twisted Chair Pose:

1. From the chair pose, pull your hands to your chest in prayer position

2. Simultaneously slide your shoulder blades down

3. Twist from the navel towards the right side and twist your left elbow across the right knee

4. Press the left elbow against the outer edge of the right knee

5. Stay in the pose for 2 counts

After the twisted pose on the right side, bring arms back to center and come back to the chair pose, hold for 2 counts and then twist to the left side, come back to the chair pose - this completes one round

Total 8 rounds

Dolphin To Forearm Plank...15 To 20 Rounds

Tabletop Pose

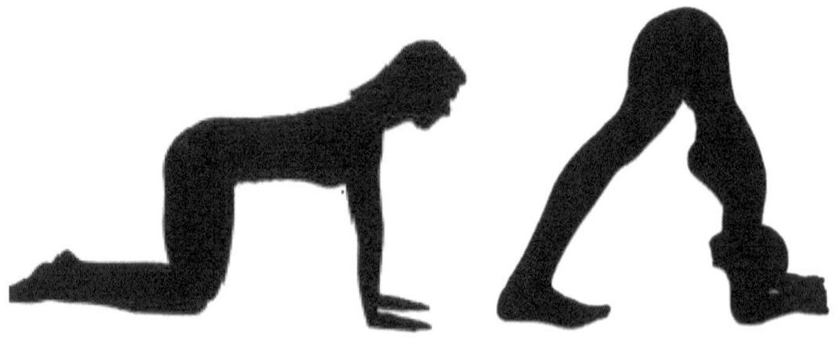

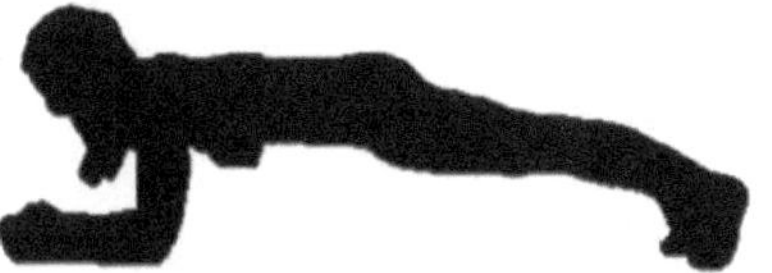

1. Come on your fours with hands under the shoulders and knees under the hips. Fingers are facing forward and feet in line with the knees

2. The torso is parallel to the mat

3. To maintain balance keep distance between palms the same as the distance between knees

4. Engage the abs and keep a natural spine - Spine being in one line between the tail bone and crown of the head

5. Gaze down between the palms

Dolphin Pose

1. From tabletop pose, put your forearms down, bring feet on toes and raise hips upwards towards the roof

2. The palms are shoulder-width apart

3. Press the palms, forearms, and fingers; and raise hips up and back

4. The feet are hip-width apart

5. The back remains straight and if possible press the heels down

6. The neck and shoulders are soft

7. Lower your head down and try to rest the forehead on the mat. If it is not possible, then hang head and neck freely between the shoulders - gazing at the mat below

8. Interlace fingers with palms together

9. Hold the pose for 2 counts

Forearm Plank

1. To come out of the dolphin pose, press your forearms and elbows, and lengthening your spine, dive forward

2. Both the legs are straight, and alongside each other

3. Both the knees are straight, up and off the mat

4. Engage abs and keep the spine straight and neutral

5. Neck remains long

6. The body remains in one line from the top of the head down to your heels

7. The body is parallel to the mat

8. Gaze down at the mat

9. Stay in pose for 2 counts

Dive up lifting hips up and back

Get back into dolphin pose

This completes one round

Complete 20 to 25 rounds

Tree Pose To Crescent Lunge Twist

Tree Pose

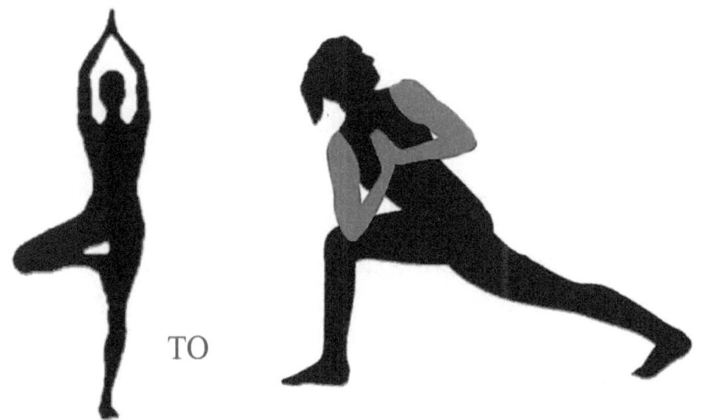

1. Begin in tadasana

2. Shift your weight on left foot and ground on four corners of the left foot

3. Bend your right knee

4. Clasp for your right ankle and place right foot on the inside of your left leg either above the knee or below the knee

5. The right knee points out to the side

6. If you can place the foot on the left inner thigh, then press the foot on to the thigh and the thigh on the foot

7. The same applies if you have placed your left foot below the knee i.e. press the foot onto the calf and the calf onto the foot

8. Engage your core, squeeze your hip muscles, lengthen your spine and keep chin raised up (chin in and back)

9. Keep the shoulder and neck muscles soft

10. Raise your arms straight upwards; and besides your ears

11. Keeping the arms shoulder width apart, join palms together

12. Stay in the pose for 2 counts

Bring arms back down and pull your hands to the chest in prayer position.

Get into Crescent lunge twist

Crescent Lunge Twist

1. Pull your left leg backward

2. Engage your left quad (inner thighs) and lift the left knee cap upwards

3. The right knee remains directly over the ankle or slightly behind the ankle

4. Initiate twist at the naval and twist to the right side

5. Twist your left elbow across the right knee and press the left elbow against the outer edge of the right knee

6. Join palms of both hands in a prayer position and keep the right elbow lifted upwards

7. Engage core and keep your upper body lifted. The spine remains straight and lengthened

8. Gaze up and remain in the pose for 2 counts

9. Come out of the pose and twist back and bring both palms down beside your feet and get into halfway lift pose

10. Raise up to tadasana

Repeat both the poses with the other leg and you complete one round.

Complete 6 to 8 rounds

Cobra Pose To Down Dog Pose

Cobra Pose

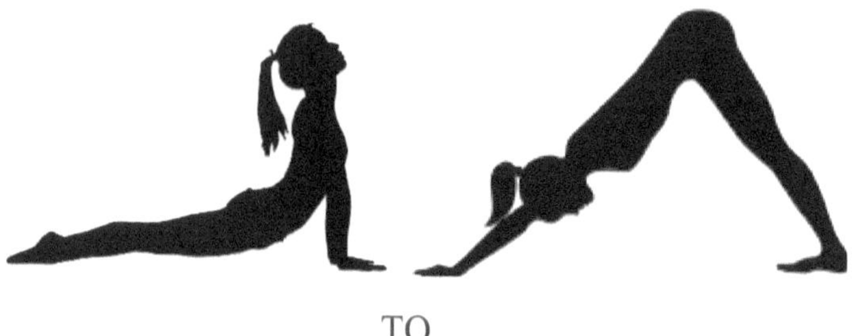

TO

1. Begin with lying on the abdomen

2. Legs are stretched with the toes touching the mat

3. Chin is on the mat

4. Bring your palms beside your armpits

5. Pressing the hips on the mat, gently raise your chest up

6. Press shoulders down and back, and arch your spine evenly

7. Bend backward as much as you can and gaze up

8. The hips have to remain planted onto the mat and navel off the mat

9. Soften neck and shoulders and gaze straight

10. Be in the pose for 2 counts

11. Get into down dog

Down Dog

1. Lower your head and chest down to the mat from cobra

2. Bring the feet on your toes

3. Engage your core muscles and applying pressure on your palms and balls of your feet raise your hips up to the roof

4. Push shoulders inwards between the arms so that the inside of your arms are aligned in line with the ears

5. The feet are hip distance apart

6. Adjust feet - probably bring them a little inwards and see that the heels are down on the mat

7. Externally rotate (backward rotation) the shoulders and spread the shoulder blades wide

8. Let the arms be wide - shoulder-distance

9. Straighten your legs and keep lifting hip up coming into an upside-down "V" shape

10. Relax your head between your arms, push your body in and look inwards towards your knees

11. Stay in the pose for 2 counts

12. Taking weight on your palms, bring your feet on the tip of your toes and lift hip upwards

13. Arching your spine inwards, pull your body forward and gently lower yourself onto your abs

14. Get back into cobra

This is one round

Complete 15 to 20 rounds

Warrior 1 To Warrior 3

Warrior One

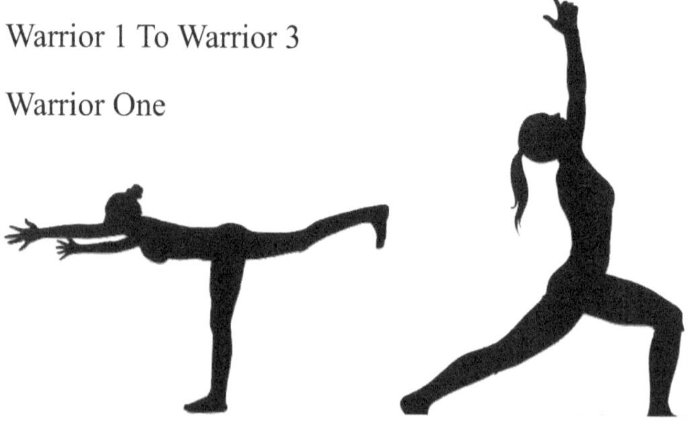

1. Begin in tadasana

2. Extend left foot backward

3. The left leg behind remains straight and both the feet are flat on the mat

4. The right leg in the front is bent at 90 degrees angle at the knee and the knee is stacked over the ankle or slightly behind but not in front of the ankle

5. The ankle of both the legs stay in a line

6. The front thigh remains parallel to the mat (this is possible if you can square the hips)

7. Try and distribute weight evenly on four corners of both feet

8. Pull the shoulders away from the ears and lift the arms up keeping neck and spine long. interlace fingers

9. Gaze at the interlaced fingers

10. Stay in the pose for 2 counts

11. Get into warrior 3

Warrior 3

1. Open arms and bring your arms down beside your body

2. Lowering your torso down, slowly lift up the left leg drawing your tummy to the spine

3. Keep lowering the torso and head and bring your body parallel to the ground

4. Simultaneously extend arms forward

5. Arms remain straight and engaged

6. Micro bend the right knee

7. Flex the lifted foot and actively engage it. Push through heel as though you are pushing the wall

8. Create length through the neck by gazing ahead of you downwards (to the top of the mat)

9. Keep your spine long and square your hips evenly to the ground

10. If you are a beginner you can try this pose by keeping your hands on the wall or your hips

11. You can even avoid taking the lifted leg high

12. Stay in the pose for 2 counts

13. Bring your left leg down and arms beside the body

14. Bring the left foot forward beside the right foot

15. Extend right foot backward and repeat the above

16. This completes one round

17. Complete 10 to 15 rounds each side

Warrior 2 To Star Pose To Warrior 2 To Star Pose

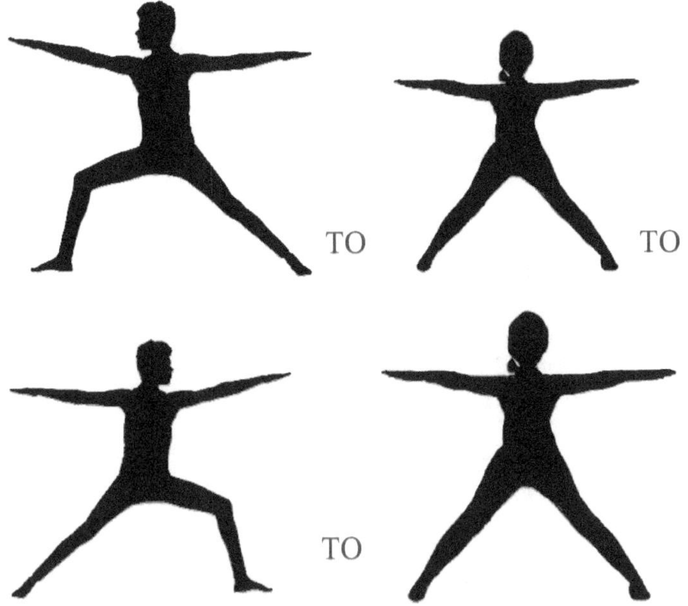

1. Begin in tadasana

2. From tadasana extend left foot backward

3. Bend the right leg until the right knee is over the ankle and 90 degrees angle to the thigh (if hips can be kept squared)

4. The leg behind (left leg) is straight

5. The heels are in a line and the heel of the back foot is pointing back

6. The navel is facing forward and is in line with the shoulders

7. Shoulders away from the ears and arms extend out in line with the shoulders

8. The arms remain parallel to the mat

9. Gaze to the front fingers/arms

10. Be in the pose for 2 counts

11. Get into star pose

Star Pose

1. Straighten your front leg (right leg)

2. Turn both your feet out and face forward

3. Raise both your arms in line with your shoulders

4. Stay for two counts and back to warrior 2 pose on the other side

Warrior 2 On The Left Side

1. Bend your left leg and turn towards your bent left leg

2. The left knee is over the ankle and 90 degrees angle to the thigh (if hips can be kept squared)

3. The leg behind (right leg) is straight

4. The rest same as mentioned above - points 5 to 9

5. Stay in the pose for 2 counts

6. Get into star pose

Stay in star pose for 2 counts and this completes one round

Complete 8 to 10 rounds each side

Seated Spinal Twist To Down Dog Splits

Seated Spinal Twist

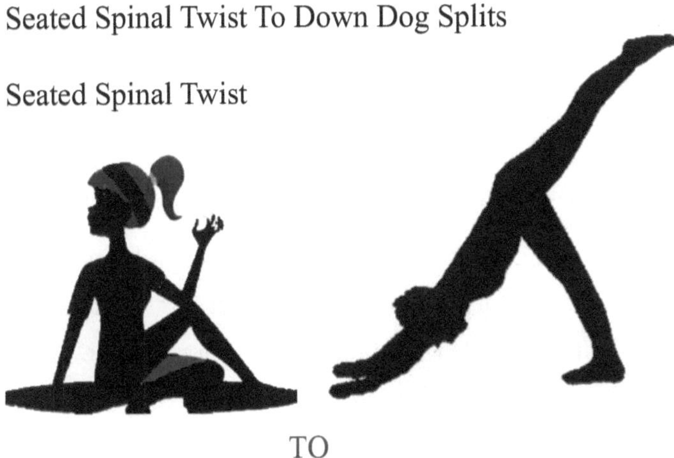

TO

1. Begin in long sitting

2. Fold your right leg and bring the right ankle close to the left buttocks

3. Hold the right ankle and pull the right foot close to the left hip such that right heel touches the left hip

4. The outside edge of the right foot, the ankle and the pinky toe are all pressed into the mat

5. Fold your left leg, hold the left foot and bring it next to the outside of the right thigh and place it in such a way that the left shin remains perpendicular to the mat

6. Your torso is straight with chin raised up

7. Your left arm is straight beside your hip with the palm facing downwards and fingertips facing forward

8. Twist from your navel towards the left side

9. Bring your right arm towards the left and twist more to place the right upper arm in front of the outside of the left knee. If possible press the right armpit into your left knee

10. Straightening your right arm slightly try and grab your left ankle.

11. Expand your chest, swing your left arm behind your back and roll over the middle back with palms facing out and fingertips over the right waist

12. Turn your head towards the left and gaze over the left shoulder

13. Breathe normally, keep your shoulders and neck relaxed and keep twisting the torso more inch by inch

14. Stay for 2 counts

15. Get into downward dog pose

Down Dog Pose

1. Release arms and return to the starting position

2. Fold both legs such that both the knees face towards the right and the left thigh is on the right thigh, the left foot on the right foot

3. Twist from navel towards the right side bringing both arms to the right side and placing the palms close to the outer side of the right thigh. Fingers face forward

4. Raise hips and torso and come on your fours

5. Kneel on all fours with hips over your knees and shoulders over your elbows

6. Let the arms be wide - shoulder-distance

7. Lift hip up, straighten your legs, lower your heels towards the ground and come into an upside-down "V" shape

Down Dog Splits

1. Relax your head between your arms, push your body in and look inwards towards your knees

2. Raise right foot up to the roof and root the left foot into the mat

3. Stay for one count

4. Bring leg back to position

5. Raise left foot up to the roof and root the right foot into the mat

6. Bring leg back to position

7. Fold legs and sit down and come back to long sitting

8. Fold the left leg and bring the left ankle close to the right buttocks

9. Repeat the same as 3 to 14 instructions as in Seated spinal twist

10. Get into one-legged down dog

11. After raising each leg into one-legged down dog, get back to the starting position (long sitting)

This completes one round

Complete 6 to 8 rounds each side

If you have knee pain -rather than folding one leg and bringing the heel to the hip, keep it straight out in front of you

THIS COMPLETES MODULE 1

Module 2

Tadasana To Forward Bend To Boat

Forward Bend Pose

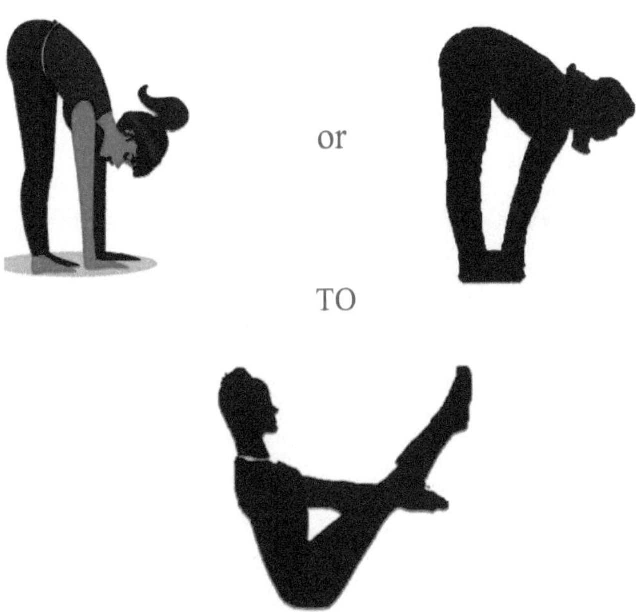

1. Begin in tadasana

2. Shoulders away from the ears (by rotating the shoulders outward)

3. Open the chest by drawing the shoulder blades down towards the spine

4. Ensure to keep a straight back

5. Distribute weight equally on four corners of your feet

6. Slowly bend down from your hips keeping them in line with the heels

7. As you bend engage your core, elongate neck in line with the spine, and bring your chest to thighs

8. Do not curl the neck and see that the crown of your head faces the mat

9. Reach for your ankles or your shin or cup your fingers and place the tips on the mat

10. Alternatively, bend the knees or place the palms on blocks to help reach the ground.

11. You can bend your knees slightly and hold onto your shins to lessen the stretch

12. Stay in the pose for 2 counts

13. Get into boat pose

Boat Pose

1. In forward bend pose, fold your legs and gently bend your knees and bring your hips down on the mat

2. The knees are facing the roof and the feet are flat on the mat

3. Release arms and bring them to the side of your hips

4. Come on your sit bones (2 bones at the bottom of your pelvis, one on each side)

5. Keep your spine straight and neck long

6. Leaning back a little, straighten and raise the folded legs up

7. The shins are parallel to the mat

8. Engage your abs, open your chest and keep lengthening your torso

9. Stay in the pose for 2 counts

10. Get back into standing forward fold

11. This completes one round

To get back to forward fold - fold the legs and bring feet flat on the mat. Bring arms back to the sides of the hips with palms on the mat. Lift hips and straighten the legs. Simultaneously bend torso down to get back to forward fold

Pigeon Stretch To Fish Pose

Pigeon Stretch

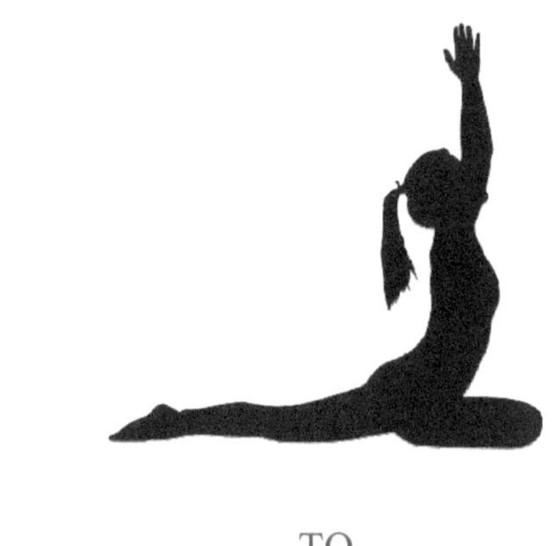

TO

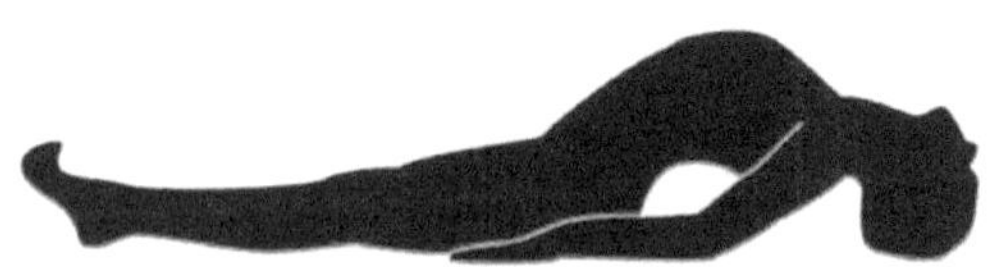

1. Begin from the tabletop pose (explained in module 1, exercise 2)

2. Bring your right knee close to your right wrist

3. Hold the right ankle with your left hand and fold it so that the right soles face on the left side and the right knee points to the right

4. Gently slide the left leg straight behind, with the front of your left foot on the mat and the heel pointing the roof

5. If possible adjust the right leg in such a way that the right shins are parallel to the front of your mat and the right ankle is somewhere in front of the left hip

6. Scissor and square your hips

7. The arms are straight beside the hips with palms facing down

8. Gently press palms on the mat, engage your abs, lengthen your spine and your torso and open your chest

9. Raise your arms up, besides the ears and bring palms in prayer position

10. Lengthen your torso and look up at the palms opening the chest a little more

11. Stay in the pose for 2 counts and then get into the fish pose

Fish Pose

1. To come out of the pigeon pose, bring arms down beside your hips, raise hips and push back with the support of your arms and move the leg back and get back to tabletop pose

2. From tabletop, bring your hips down and simultaneously fold both legs either to the left or to the right - the legs are one over the other

3. Bring your arms beside your hips

4. Fold both arms at the elbow, unfold legs and strengthen them and get into the long sitting pose

5. Bending your torso and head back, gently put forearms down and put slight weight onto your elbows

6. Lower your back down and come into a supine pose

7. Your arms rest beside your sides and legs are extended and close to each other. Palms are facing down

8. Bring the palms under the hips, press the elbows lightly and raise your chest and head off the mat

9. Raise chest more and gently bring the crown of your head on the mat, keeping your toes pointed backwards

10. Ensure there is no pressure on your head and neck

11. Be in the pose for 2 counts

12. Get back to pigeon pose

To come out of the fish pose, release head and torso to the mat and come back to supine pose. Raise up and sit up folding both legs together to any one side. Get into the tabletop pose and then into pigeon with the other leg. from pigeon you get into the fish pose and back to supine and on fours. This completes one round. Complete 4 to 6 rounds

Plank Variation Push-Ups To Side Plank Pose

Plank Variation Push-Ups

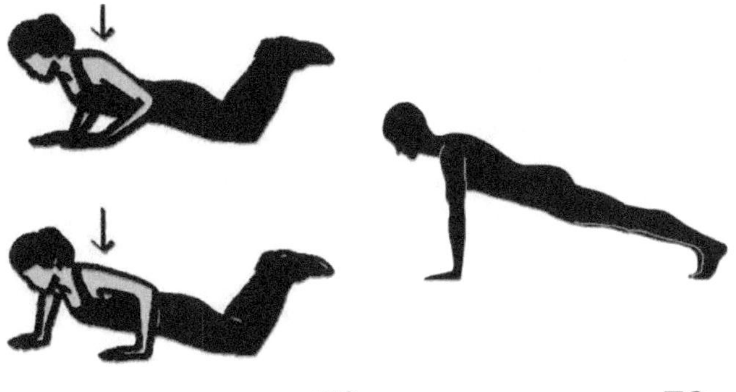

TO   TO

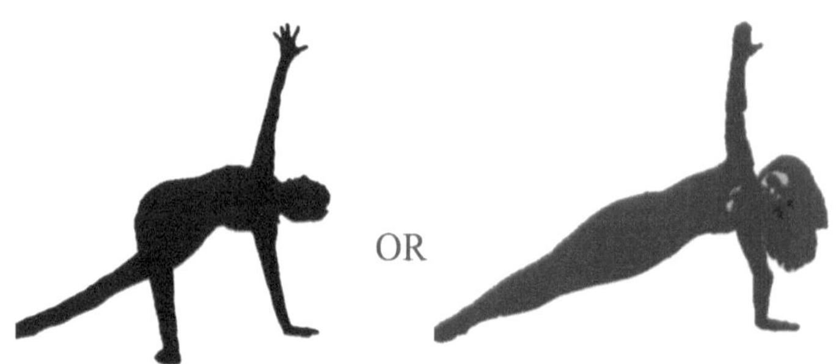

1. Begin in tabletop position with your hand and knees in a high push up position

2. The arms are a little more outside your shoulder width. Keep the palms on the mat a little forward than the shoulders

3. Raise both your lower limbs up till they are perpendicular to the thighs and soles of the feet face the roof

4. Cross your feet at the ankles

5. Engage your abs and keep your spine neutral

6. Gently lower your torso and head by bending 90 degrees angle at the elbows (if 90 degrees angle is not possible, go up to a comfortable position)

7. Push the elbows back and not out

8. Keep legs together while you do the push-up and maintain their stability

9. Push back up, by straightening your arms. Keep your shoulders, neck, and elbows soft

10. Repeat 4 times and then get into plank

Plank

1. Extend the right leg straight back, with the foot on your toes. Extend the left leg too and place it alongside the right foot

2. Both the legs are straight, up, with the knees off the mat

3. Keep your spine and neck long

4. Distribute weight equally on your toes and palms

5. The body remains in one line from the top of the head down to your heels

6. The body is parallel to the mat

7. The arms are directly underneath your shoulders

8. Get into side plank pose

Side Plank

1. In the plank pose, twist to the right side and shift your weight to the right side of the body - mainly the right arm and the outer edge of the feet

2. Roll on to the outer edge of the right foot

3. Bring the left leg over the right leg

4. Both the legs are extended with the left leg on the top of the right leg

5. Press gently the right-hand palm, mainly the arch of the palm and not the base

6. Raise the left arm up towards the roof

7. Keep core muscles engaged and maintain a straight body

8. Keep shoulders stacked on one top of the other

9. Lift bottom chest high and firm the bottom shoulder into the ribs

10. If you do not have the strength to perform this pose with right alignment, then you can get into the modified side plank pose until you can support your body weight correctly

Modified Side Plank

1. When you twist to the right side - extend the right leg and roll on to the outer edge of the right foot

2. Bend the left knee and bring your left foot in front of your right knee

3. The toes of the left foot point forward

4. Stack your shoulders, press the right palm gently and raise the left arm up

5. Press the four corners of the left foot and raise hips higher

6. Stay for 2 counts and get back to plank variation

Repeat with the other leg, on the other side - for a side plank. This completes one round. Complete 10 rounds each side

Malasana To Plank To Malasana

Malasana

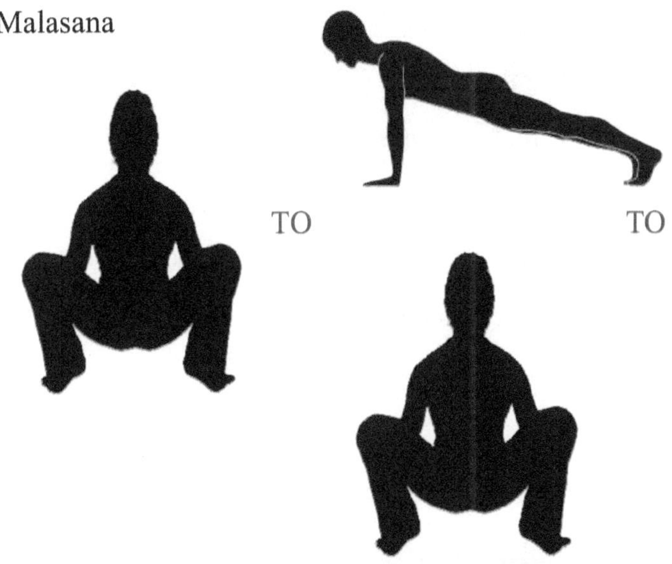

1. Begin in Tadasana

2. Place legs outside of hips and point toes slightly out

3. Press down and drop your hip as far down as comfortable

4. See that the knees point in the direction as the toes. If your hips are tight the knees might turn inwards. Therefore, listen to your body and do not try to exceed your limits

5. If your heels lift up its fine, if you can, try to keep them down but do not force them down

6. Once down and comfortable, press palms together near the chest

7. Keep lengthening your spine

8. Press the inside of the knees with the elbows to widen the knees and to open up the hips more

9. If your heels are close to touching the mat, widen your stance to see if they touch

10. If they do not touch it is fine to raise them

11. Now open up your ankles, your hips and relax

12. As there is no one size fits all squat, keep adjusting

your stance width or your elbow placement till you are comfortable in the pose

13. Stay in the pose for 2 counts

14. Get into plank pose

Plank Pose

1. Open your palms and place them on the mat in between the feet

2. If you can, jump to plank pose and if you cannot jump, extend the right leg straight back with the foot on your toes and then extend the left leg too and place it alongside the right foot

3. Both the legs are straight and up with the knees off the mat

4. Keep your spine and neck long

5. Distribute weight equally on your toes and palms

6. The body remains in one line from the top of the head down to your heels

7. The body is parallel to the mat

8. The arms are directly underneath your shoulders

9. Stay in the pose for 2 counts and get back to malasana

10. This completes one round

11. Complete 15 to 20 repetitions

To get back to malasana from plank, you can either jump back or if not extend one leg forward and then the other leg and get into the pose

Revolved Side Angle Pose To Reverse Warrior Pose

Revolved Side Angle

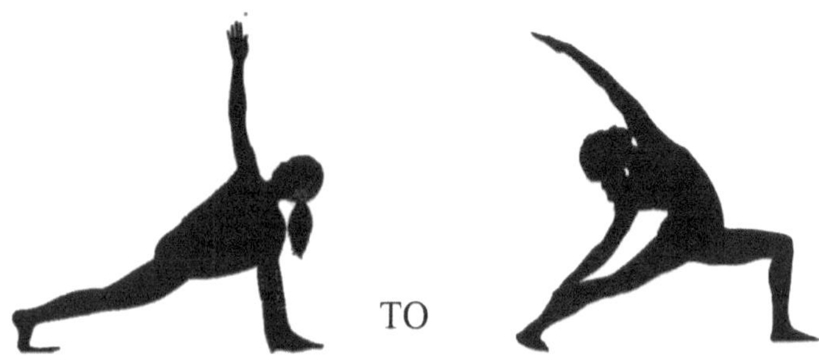

1. Begin in tadasana

2. Slowly bend down from your hips keeping them in line with the heels

3. As you bend engage your core, elongate neck in line with the spine and bring your chest to thighs

4. The crown of your head faces the mat

5. Place the palms on the mat - bending the knees slightly

6. Gaze forward

7. Extend the left leg straight behind and engage the left thigh muscles

8. Keep the right leg bent in the front with the right knee stacked over the right ankle or slightly behind. The right thigh makes a 90 degrees angle with the right calf and is parallel to the mat

9. You are in a high lunge position, wherein both your heels are in line with each other.

10. Bring your left palm close to the outer side of your right foot, twist your torso and your head towards the right side and lift up the right arm upwards besides your right ear. The right arm is perpendicular to your right side

11. Press the left hand gently into the mat such that the back of your left armpit is against the outside of your right knee.

12. Lengthen the right side of your body all the way from your right foot to your right fingertips

13. Keep your shoulders soft

14. Expand your chest and pull it slightly back such that your chest, hips, and right leg all stay in one line

15. Stay in the pose for 2 counts and then get into reverse warrior

Reverse Warrior

1. To come out of the revolved side angle pose, bring the right palm down and place it beside the left foot

2. Lift torso up and straighten your spine straight. Neck and shoulder muscles remain relaxed and the spine is lengthened. Bring arms beside your body

3. Gently get into a backbend and place the left hand on the back of the left thigh and glide down till body permits

4. Raise the right arm up towards the ceiling and reach the fingers away from each other

5. Keep the right knee bent and sink the right feet into the mat

6. Lengthen the sides of your torso

7. If neck permits turn your gaze towards the fingertips of your right arm

8. Stay in the pose for 2 counts

9. To come out of the pose, unfold your back and bring arms to the sides of the torso. Bend torso in a forward fold, place palms down on the mat on either side of the right foot and get into a high lunge pose

10. Repeat on the other side by getting into revolved side angle pose first and then into reverse warrior pose

11. This completes one round

12. Complete 6 to 8 rounds on both sides

Chair To Warrior 1 And Warrior Dips And Back To Chair

Chair Pose

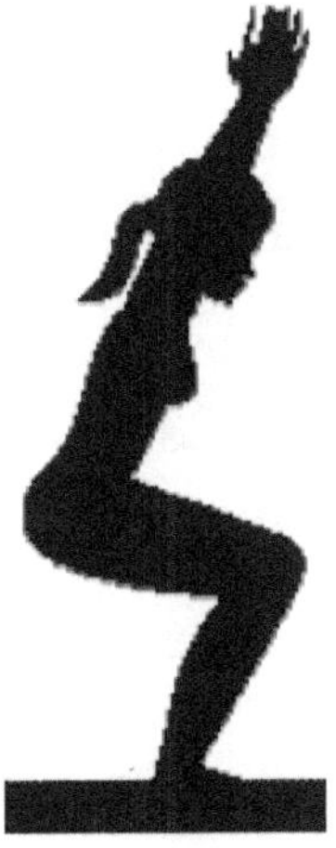

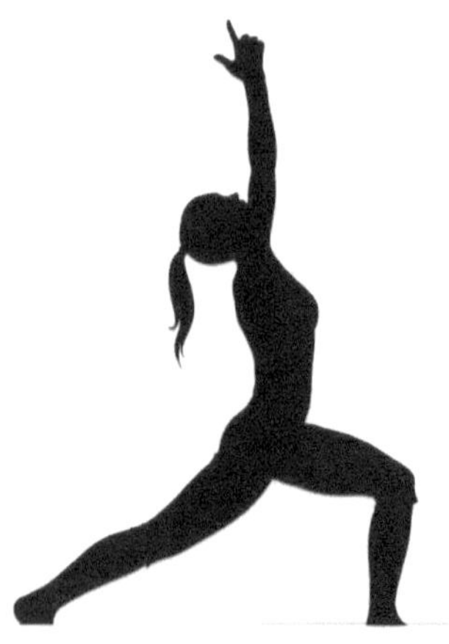 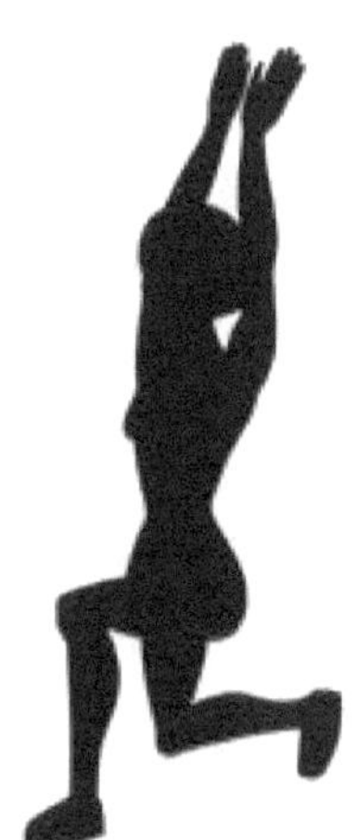

1. As described in module 1, exercise number 1, get into chair pose

2. Stay in the pose for 2 counts

3. Get into warrior 1

Warrior 1

1. To get into warrior 1 from chair pose, extend your left leg straight behind.

2. Repeat as described in module 1, exercise number 5, points 3 to 9

3. Do 5 dips in this pose...

Warrior 1 Dips

1. In warrior 1 pose, gently lower your rear knee

(the left knee) down till your body permits (you can even touch the mat if possible)

2. As you dip down push your hips slightly forward

3. Arms remain stretched upwards

4. Stand up back to warrior 1 pose

5. Repeat this action 5 times and get back to chair pose

To Get Back To Chair Pose From Warrior 1

1. Bring arms down to the sides of the body

2. Bend forward and place palms down on the mat on either side of the right foot

3. Bring the left foot back to the front beside the right foot

4. Get into half forward fold

5. Get into chair pose

6. Repeat with the other leg

7. This completes one round

8. Complete 5 rounds with each leg

Bridge Pose To Konasana

Bridge Pose

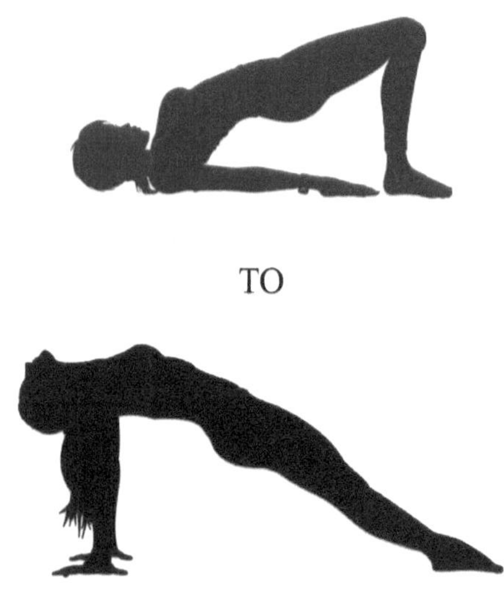

TO

1. Begin in a supine position

2. Fold your legs at the knees with your feet flat on the mat and hip-distance away

3. Stack your knees and heels

4. Arms are straight beside your body with palms facing down

5. Bring the feet close to your buttocks

6. Broaden your collar bones and lift your chest up.

7. Squeeze your buttocks and lift them away from the floor

8. Gently press the center of your head onto the mat

9. Squeeze your buttocks and keep your lower back safe

10. Slowly move your chin away from the chest so that there is a slight gap between your neck and the mat

11. Drive your hip more up and forward

12. The inner edges of the feet are parallel to each other

13. Gaze up

14. Stay in the pose for 2 counts

15. Gently lower your hips and torso down

16. Get into reverse plank pose

Reverse Plank Pose

1. After you lower down from bridge pose, fold your legs to bring the knees to the chest

2. Hold the folded legs with both your arms and hug your knees

3. Roll up

4. Straighten your legs and sit in long position - legs straight, feet together and heels on the mat.

5. Arms on the ground on either side of the body with fingers pointing forward

6. Push up and lift your hips, torso, and head, by gently pressing the heels and arms on the mat

7. Keep lifting until you form a straight line from head to toes

8. Keep your abs and glutes engaged

9. Do not droop and keep arms and legs straight

10. Soften shoulders and neck

11. Gaze straight

12. Stay in the pose for 2 counts

13. Lower your body down and sleep on your back

14. This completes one round

15. Complete 10 rounds

When cardio and yoga asanas are blended together harmoniously, they end up burning calories at a much higher rate and not only tones or sculpt your body but helps in improving your balance, flexibility, endurance, and posture.

The above 20 to 30 - minute cardio yoga workout modules do not need any equipment other than a mat and your body weight. The module targets almost all your muscle groups - the glutes, abdominal core, shoulders, quads, hamstrings, triceps and biceps, and most important - your back. Have super fun with these cardio, strength and flexibility moves; all in one workout.

Avoid injuries and muscle imbalances

Stretch, Sweat, and feel your heart beating within your chest

Live your best life to the absolute fullest!

CHAPTER 6

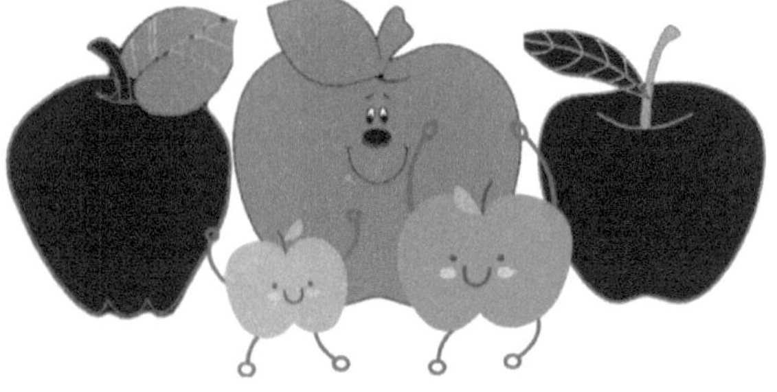

6. CAN WE COMPARE APPLES TO APPLES

Yogalates – A fusion of yoga and pilates

The other day, I was having lunch with one of my friends and her young daughter. We were generally discussing about health, fitness, diet etc., when somewhere in between the subject of yoga came up. My friend's daughter immediately interrupted and said, "Ma'am, not yoga please! You cannot call it a workout".

I was neither shocked nor disturbed on hearing this, because this is how 80% of youngsters feel. Instead, I replied, "Ohh, why dear? Then, according to you what makes for a good workout?"

She replied, "Something that is challenging, something that keeps you moving and something that brings all the liquid (sweat) from the body onto the clothes in 20 to 30 minutes. Sitting for an hour in a yoga class is absolute torture for me!"

Now, I agree with the movement and time factors, but I disagree with the sweat part of the conversation :)

Sweating has never been a reliable indicator for a hard workout. There are a list of factors that determine how much you sweat during exercise viz. gender, age, humidity, genetics, metabolic rate, etc

Movement and time factor are acceptable parameters as they are common personality traits found in today's generation. Personalities matter in every industry, and yoga is no different. Therefore, to keep up with today's anxious and restless generation, it was important for me to integrate my yoga classes with a style that complements and balances their personality.

Thus, along with incorporating asanas with cardio, I also brought Pilates to my yoga mat. Their bodies needed variety, so I tried mixing up the two beautiful philosophies of yoga and Pilates, and voila! Yogalates was born!

Yogalates is a fusion of two perspectives of moves or asanas, which are almost the same but differ in style. They both are mind-body practices with a focus on breath, alignment, balance, strength, and flexibility. What is interesting about pilates is, you hold a pose for a very small count and repeat it for 5 to 10 counts (all this done with focus, precision, and total control). Once done, you get into a completely new move. The movement, grace, and creativity totally appeals to young practitioners and they happily roll over their mats for it.

I had to get trained in Pilates and therefore joined a course in the same. The classes were as amazing as yoga and were yet specifically different. Pilates helped me work with my spine in a better way and corrected the spinal misalignments caused after my road accident. I learned the art of supporting my movements with my core muscles and therefore put less stress on my back. Engaging distinct muscles in Pilates has helped in strengthening my yoga flows and stretching of the muscles in yoga has aided me in relaxing the worked-out muscles in Pilates. The techniques of these two disciplines complement each other and convert into an irrefutable workout combo. I would like to mention here that the fusion of pilates and yoga has helped my yoginis build a strong core and advance gracefully into poses that they felt were tougher to get into before - all this done with a safe back and, of course, NO DRAMA.

It's time now to grab the mat and start our journey to health with something that is kind to our body, prevents injuries and is a rewarding complement to our yoga practice.

Before we head over to our yogalates workout day (keep one day of your week for this workout to add variety and spice) let's talk about:

Neutral spine and the 6 basic principles of pilates

Neutral Spine

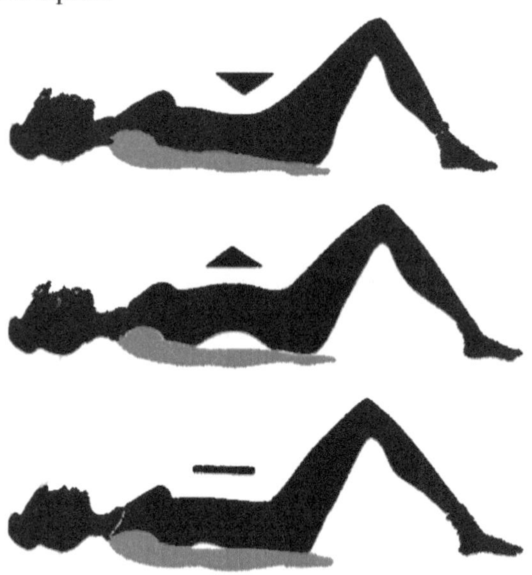

The strongest position for your spine to be in is the 'neutral spine position'. It is the position that cushions your back and there is the least stress on the disks.

Finding a neutral spine is crucial in pilates. It's all about the presence and alignment of the three natural curves of the spine - the lumbar, thoracic and cervical. The cervical spine (neck) and lumbar (lower back) curves gently inwards and the thoracic(middle) curves gently outwards

How to find?

Lie on your back with your legs bent, feet flat on the mat and arms at your sides.

Relax your jaw, neck, and shoulders

Rest the back on the mat without any effort

Breathe deeply into the sides of the rib cage and the back of your body

As you breathe out, engage abs and push the lower spine into the mat in a pelvic tuck

Exhale and release

Inhale again and now pull the lower spine up and away from the mat in a pelvic tilt. Inhale and relax

Neutral spine is in between these two positions. It is a natural slight curve of the lower spine with your abs flat

How to maintain it during exercise?

Lift up your right leg up and fold it back without moving your hips. The core and pelvis remain stable

Repeat the same with the left leg

Now do this with both your legs, again keeping the core, hips and pelvis stable. If you cannot maintain stability and want to disengage the abs then you get into a pelvic tilt or pelvic tuck. It is difficult for beginners to maintain a neutral spine as the core muscles are not developed and are weak.

The ultimate goal here is to find a favourable position of the spine that allows the lower back to stay relaxed while supine and still maintain some curvature.

Basic Principles Of Pilates

Breath: coordinate your breath with each move and this should help you focus on your movements and pushes blood to your muscles

Concentration: each move has to be done mindfully; and this helps in a healthy connection with your body and mind and you can get the best out of each exercise

Centering: bring your focus to the core or the 'powerhouse' the area from where all energy for the exercise comes from

Control: instead of focussing on speed and high intensity, focus on muscular control. This will help you maintain the correct form of your moves

Precision: focus on accuracy in performing each move, more than repeating the moves in a clumsy way

Flow: the flow should be graceful, smooth, continuous and elegant

Millions of people are ardent admirers and deep believers of these 6 principles of Pilates.

Can they be adopted by anyone?

Yes! These 6 guiding principles support any age, size, gender, shape, complicacy and intensity, and they minimize the risk of injuries and benefit one and all

As we believe in 'No Drama' and simply workout (mindfully), do not bother much about the names or the order, as they all convey the same meaning in Pilates.

So, let's get onto work

Before we start with our modules let's warm up our body and prepare the abs and the lungs for what follows later

The Hundred

Appropriate for beginners to advanced people

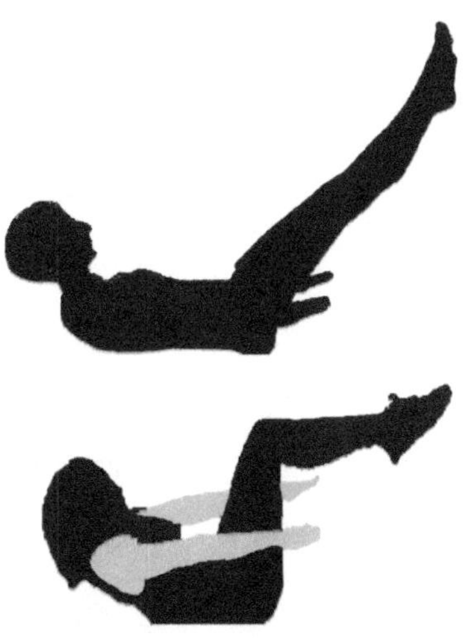

Lie on your back with a neutral spine, and arms beside your body with palms facing down

Inhale and raise up your legs to a tabletop position with your shins parallel to the mat OR extend the legs straight out towards the ceiling (as shown in the pics)

Exhale and lift up your head, neck and shoulders till the tip of your shoulder blades

The abs curl, and now lift arms up a few inches off the mat

Inhale and move arms up and down for a 5 count

Exhale and continue this moving of arms up and down for another 5 counts

Repeat this 10-count cycle till you reach 100 - these equals 100 cycles of breathing

Initially master the pilates hundred with legs in a tabletop position

The head, neck, and shoulders should remain relaxed. All the work is done by the abs alone. If you experience strain in neck or shoulders, lower your head to the mat and continue the exercise

Relax in Shavasana

Yogalates Day - Module 1 - 30 Minutes

Start your workout with 4 sets/8 rounds of Surya namaskars. Coordinate each move with breath (as explained in the chapter on Surya namaskars). The stretching's and the breath flow will warm the body enough to get the juices flowing and the heart rate up!

Relax in child pose for 10 counts

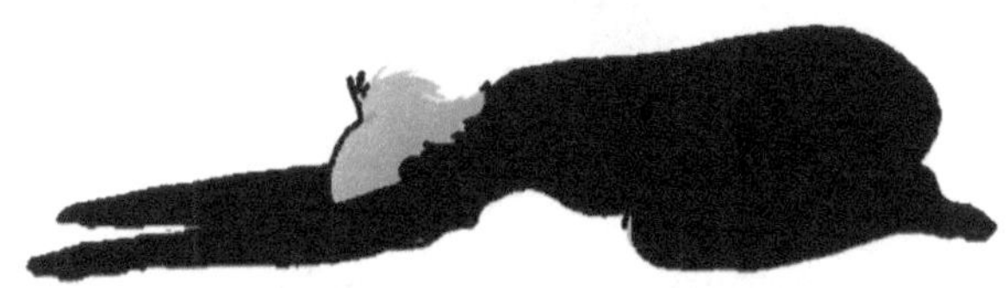

Sit in Vajrasana - sit with knees folded and place your right big toe on the left big toe. Gently press the front side of the feet on the mat and sit in the depression formed. Do not sit on your heels

You can keep the knees hips apart if you cannot join them

The palms rest on your thighs

Lower your torso and simultaneously extend arms alongside the torso

Keep lowering torso till your forehead reaches the mat

Do not curl your neck, do not curl your spine and do not raise your hips up

If your forehead cannot reach the mat it's fine; lower the torso as much as you can keeping in mind point f

Come on your fours

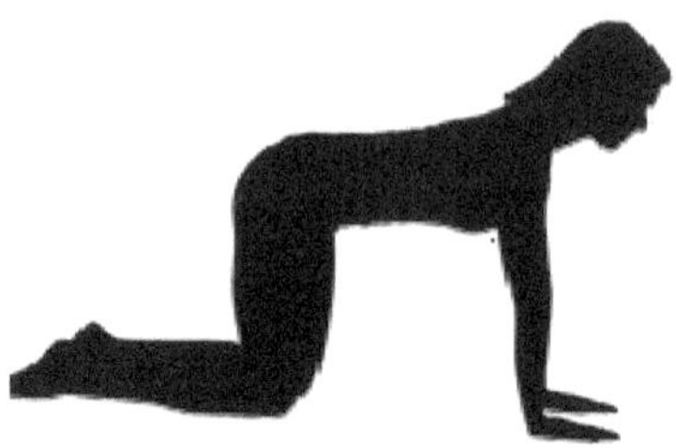

Come on your fours with hands under the shoulders and knees under the hips. Fingers are facing forward and feet in line with the knees

The torso is parallel to the mat

To maintain balance, keep distance between palms the same as the distance between knees

Engage the abs and keep a natural spine - one line between the tail bone and crown of the head

If the spine is neutral and abs are engaged then it's easy to prevent the pelvis and abdominals from collapsing towards the mat

Gaze down between the palms

Elbow to Knee Bird dog

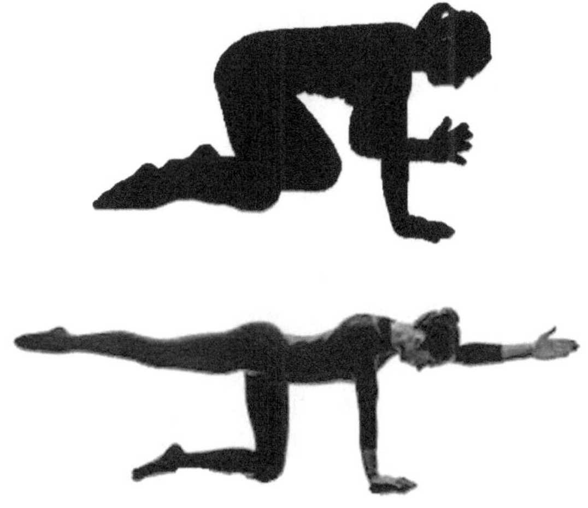

Lift your right leg 1 to 2 inches off the mat

Raise the left hand straight and forward - 1 to 2 inches off the mat

Once you gain stability to raise the arms up straight in line with your ears and extend the leg up in line with your back

Try to form one straight line from the arm to the foot

Back of the neck is in line with the spine

Keep hips squared

If lower back dips down, raise your leg as high as you can so that the back remains straight

Engage the abs and keep your hips stable

Bend elbow and bring it in and simultaneously bend the knee and bring it inwards - round your spine to bring the opposite elbow to the opposite knee

Try and make the knee and elbow touch each other

Bring back to the original position

Repeat this 10 times

Maintain the stability of the hips throughout and therefore practice it gracefully and slowly

After finishing on both sides, bring left arm back to position and extend the right leg straight back with the foot on your toes

Extend the left leg too and place it alongside the right foot

You are now in plank pose

Plank

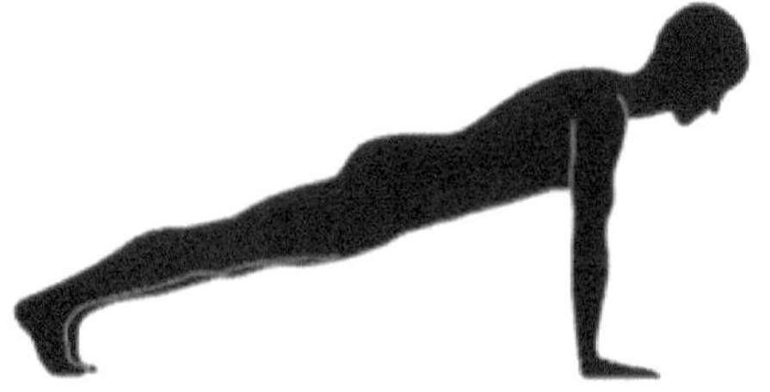

Both the knees are straight, up and off the mat

Keep your spine and neck long

Distribute weight equally on your toes and palms

The body remains in one line from the top of the head down to your heels

The body is parallel to the mat

The arms are directly underneath your shoulders

Gaze in between your palms

Tuck your legs into a crouch position

3 counts in plank and from plank get into down dog

Down dog

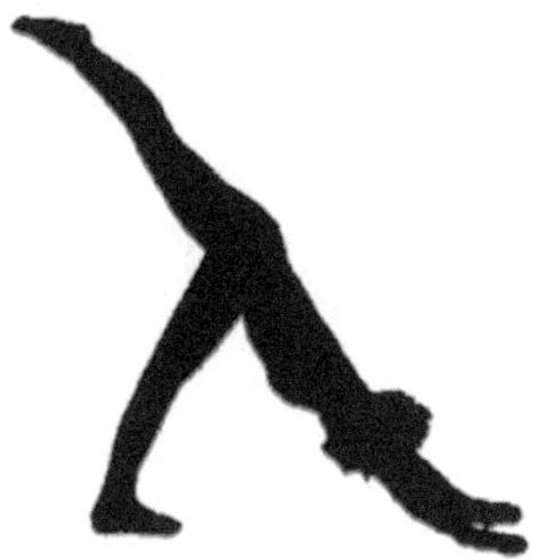

Spread the fingers wide

Externally rotate the shoulders and spread the shoulder blades wide

Let the arms be wide - shoulder-distance

Lift hip up (into an upside V shape) and simultaneously lift the right leg up

Straighten your left leg, lower your left heel towards the ground

Relax your head between your arms, push your body in and look inwards towards your knees

Fold leg and bring your right knee to your nose

The left foot raises on the toes

Knee to nose

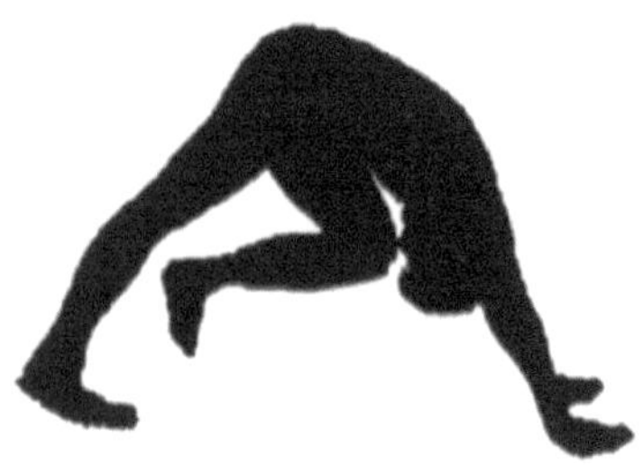

Extend leg back up

Repeat this move 3 times and on the fourth count, fold legs and bring the foot forward and place it between the palms

The left knee rests on the mat

Go for a backbend

Low lunge backbend

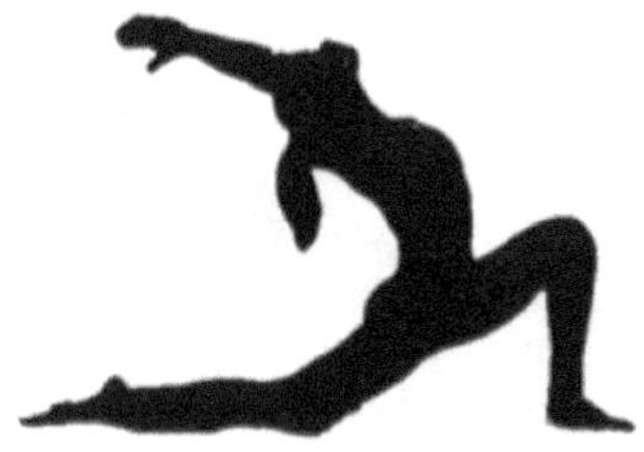

Lower your left knee onto the mat and also place the top of the left foot on the mat

Adjust the left leg till the right knee is over the heel

Lifting your torso up, raise your arms up and overhead

Gently stretch your head back and look at your hands keeping the neck long and relaxed

Bring your arms down each besides your left foot

Take the left leg behind and put it alongside the right foot and come on your fours

Repeat with the other leg from exercise 3

After repeating with both legs, get into child pose

Stay for 3 counts and then onto your all fours

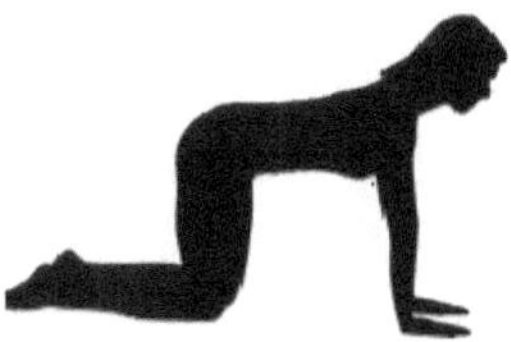

Get ready for side-lying leg raises and leg circles

Side-lying leg raising - four exercises a, b, c and d

a)

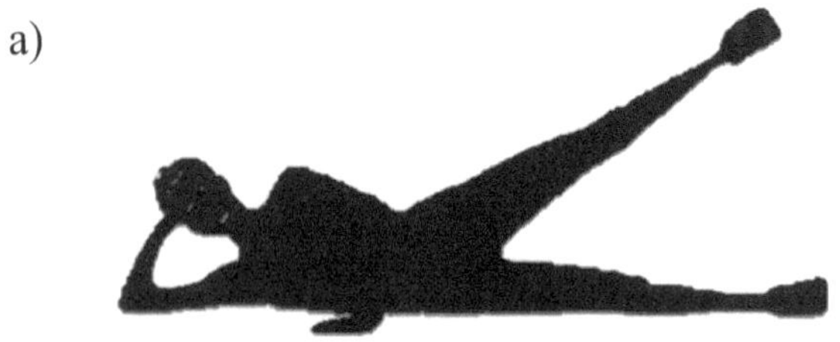

From on all fours, shift to your right side

Focus on keeping your core engaged when you practice the below moves. This should stabilize your pelvis when you move your legs. Also, keep chest expanded and shoulder blades wide to prevent sinking of the ribcage to the mat and keeping ears away from shoulders)

You also have the option of folding the bottom leg and align the kneecap to the front of the hip

The right upper arm is in line with the shoulders and forearm supports the head

See that the ankles, knees, hips, shoulders, and ears are all aligned in one line

The inner legs are together from the sit bones to the heels

Pull your abs in and lift your left leg upwards to hip

height or little more than that (but not perpendicular to the torso)

As you lift the top leg up, take care to keep both the legs parallel

Repeat it 10 counts

Side-lying leg lifts

Lying on your right side with ankles, knees, hips, shoulders, and ears are all aligned in one line

b)

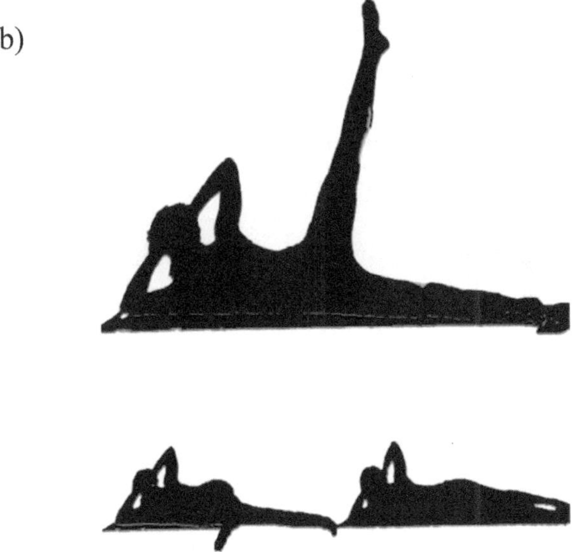

The inner legs together from the sit bones to the heels

Raise your left leg up - 90 degrees angle with the right leg

Lower it down perpendicular to the mat

If possible, try touching the big toe down on the mat

Bring leg back on top of the right leg

Repeat this move 10 reps

Side-lying leg circles

c)

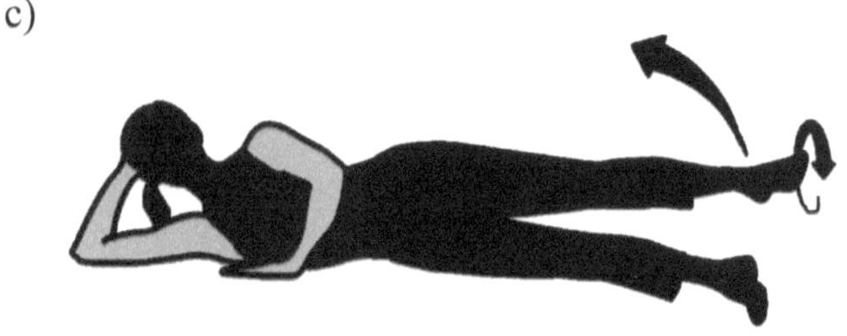

Lying on your right side with ankles, knees, hips, shoulders, and ears are all aligned in one line

The right upper arm in line with the shoulders

Support head with the right palm and wrist

Raise the left leg to hip height

Rotate the leg clockwise - keep circles small like the big toe is drawing small circles

Maintain the height of the leg - ankle around hip height

Repeat 8 clockwise rotations and similarly 8 anti-clockwise rotations with the same leg

Side-Lying Double Leg Lifts

d)

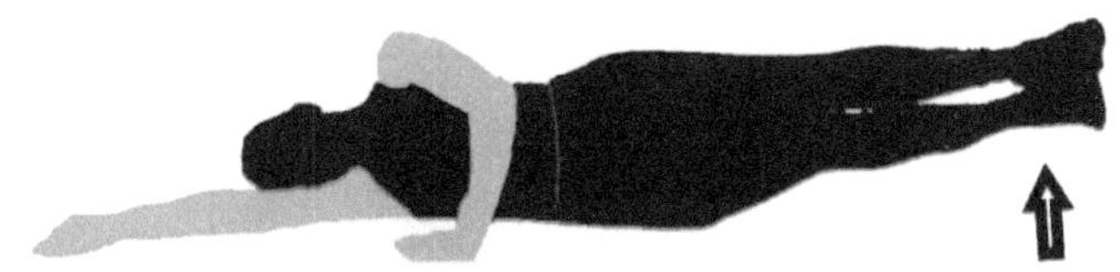

Lie on the right side with your body in a straight line as above

Extend the right arm and stack it with the knees and toes to support the head and neck

The toes are pointing forward

Place the left hand in front of the chest, mainly for light support when you raise the legs

The legs remain glued to each other during the move

Engage your abs, squeeze your inner thighs and hinging from the hips lift the legs off the mat

Hips remain stationary; therefore, lift legs only as much as possible

Repeat for 10 rounds

After you finish the 4 sets of side-lying on the right side, repeat all the 4 by side-lying on the left side

Sphinx pose

Rollover on your stomach for Sphinx pose

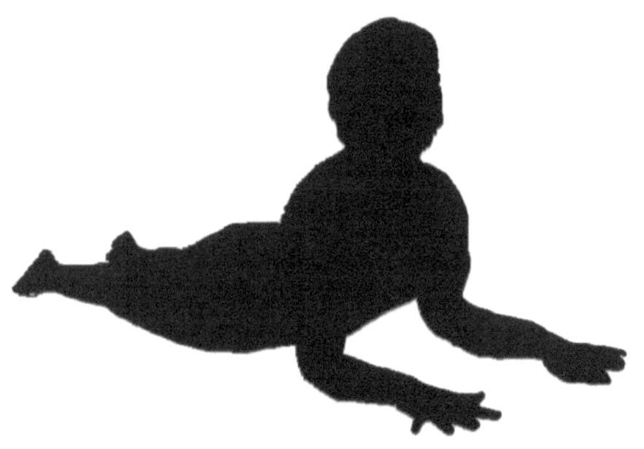

Begin with lying on the stomach with toes flat and forehead resting on the mat

Keep your legs together with heels touching each other slightly

Extend arms in the front with the forearms on the mat and palms facing downwards

Gently lift torso and head up. Keeping the navel down, gently pull torso back with the support of your forearms

Stay in the pose for 10 counts and relax

Bring your torso and head down onto the mat with forehead resting on the mat

Swan dive

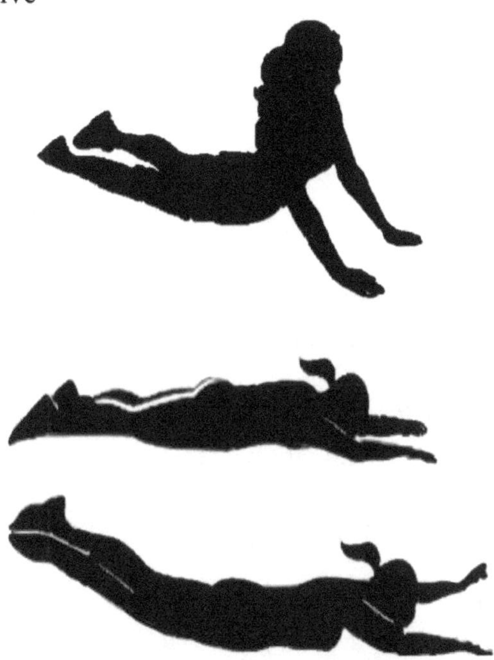

Keep legs hip-width apart

Fold arms and keep arms close to the body - the elbows are directly under the shoulder and almost near the waist

Head is resting on the forehead

Engage abs, press the forearms and hands into the mat and lift your torso, head, and navel up

Straighten arms as you raise your upper body up

Keep the neck long and the head in line with the spine

Gaze forward

Stay for 2 counts and then gently lower down, folding your elbows and with forearms besides your chest and fingers pointing forward

Repeat this move 5 counts

If all goes well then challenge yourself further by lifting both legs up - this is done as instructed below

Start with lying in a prone position with arms folded beside the body with elbows facing up

Raise your thighs up, keeping legs straight.

Squeeze your glutes and thigh muscles when you raise the legs up

As the legs come down, simultaneously straightening the arms with palms flat on the mat - raise the upper body up

You can also raise arms overhead and straight as shown in the pic

Repeat the move 6 times

Relax in a prone position and rest forehead on the mat

Next move is the swimming in pilates

Swimming in pilates

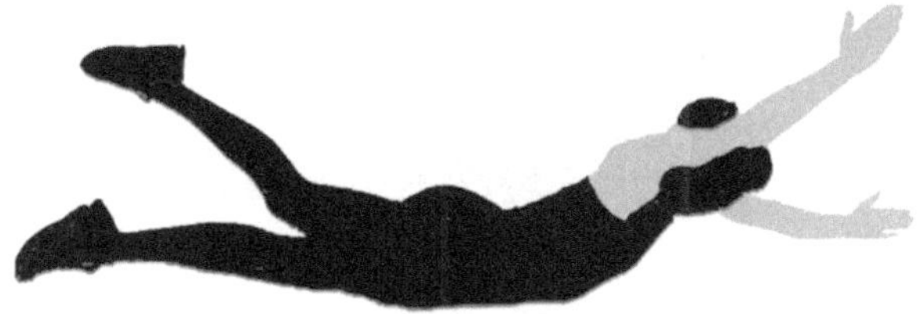

Lie on your stomach with feet together

Extend arms straight overhead with fingers pointing forward

Engage abs and lift the belly button off the floor; raise the head up keeping your spine straight

Simultaneously raise the right arm and left leg upwards

Swap arms and legs. Keep alternating right arm/left leg and left arm/right leg pulses

It should feel like swimming in a pool

Engage your core by pulling your abs in, and tightening the core muscles Keep breathing slowly

Maintain the stability of your hips and upper body

Start with one set of 10 to 15 repetitions and then when you become comfortable with the movement you can do 2 to 3 sets of 15 repetitions

Once done rest in Makarasana

Makarasana

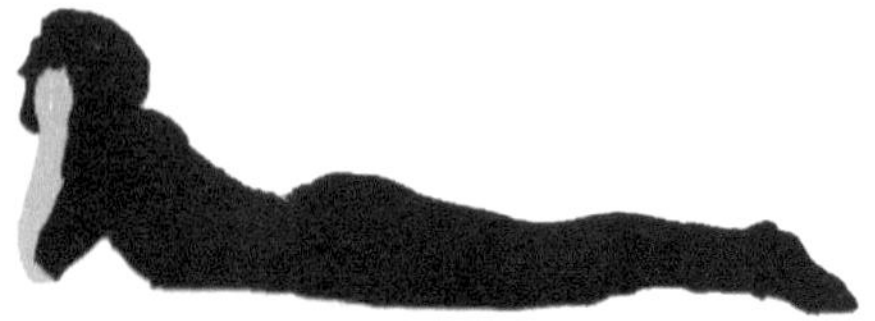

Lie down on the abdomen with chest touching the mat

Legs are apart about 2 to 3 ft

Let the toes be out to the sides, heels in and facing each other

Fold arms and lift up the head; and cup your fingers to support your head

You can also rest with the chin on the floor and arms folded and holding the opposite elbows

Relax the neck and shoulders

Close eyes and relax the whole body

Yogalates Day - Module 1I - 30 Minutes

Start with the pilates hundred 4 sets/8 rounds of Surya namaskars. Coordinate each move with breath (as explained in the chapter on Surya namaskars). The stretching's and the breath flow will warm the body enough to get the juices flowing and the heart rate up!

How to lie down on your back from tadasana without support:

Begin in tadasana

Extend right leg behind, bend the leg and put the right knee on the mat

Similarly, now extend left leg behind, bend the leg and put the left knee on the mat

Try to do the above moves without taking any support

You are now standing on your knees

Interlace your fingers and put them on the back of your head (where the head joins the neck)

Fold the legs and sit on one side of your hips. Immediately extend legs in the front and keep raising them up. Simultaneously lower your torso back till the tip of your shoulder blades

Raise both the legs and fold them into tabletop position - knees bent and shin parallel to the mat

The lower back and the middle back is on the mat and the head, neck, and shoulders are raised up till the tip of the shoulder blades

Open arms and place them besides the body

Single leg stretch

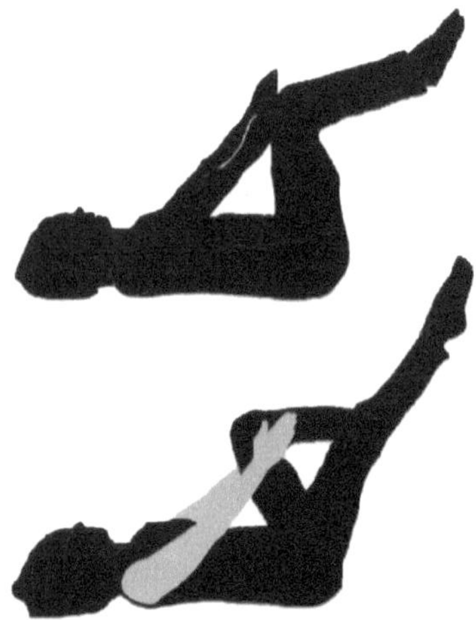

Engage your abs and extend the right leg into a 45-degree angle

The left leg remains bent

With the left arm grasp the left ankle and the right arm moves to the left knee

The shoulder and neck remain totally relaxed

Inhale and as you exhale switch legs

Now the right leg remains bent - the right arm grasps the right ankle and the left arm moves to the right knee

Inhale and switch legs again and keep repeating these moves for 10 repetitions with each leg

The movement is only with the arms and legs - the torso remains stable

Rest in Shavasana

Double leg stretch

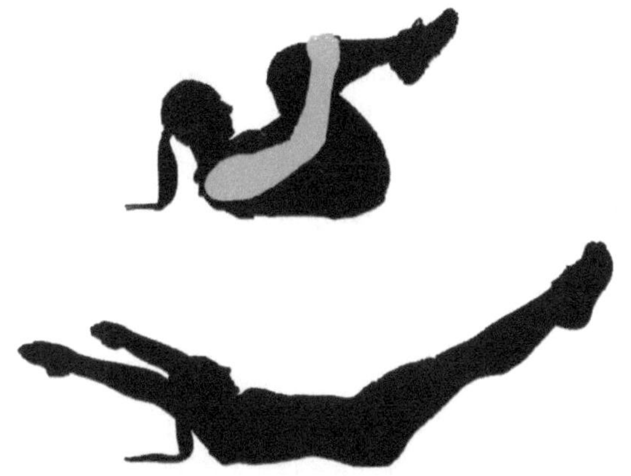

Strengthen your core with this wonderful stretch

Raise head neck shoulders till the tip of the shoulder blades

Exhale and pull your abs in, fold legs and grasp your shins and if possible, grasp your ankles

Keep your pelvis neutral and your lower back might go slightly off the mat

Bring your forehead towards your knees

Inhale and release the legs and extend them straight forward and extend arms overhead in the opposite direction (see that the ears are away from the shoulders)

Keep pulling abs in and keep lower back on the mat

Exhale and sweep arms on the sides and reach around for the legs as you fold and pull legs to the centre - you can grasp your shins and if possible, grasp your ankles

Bring forehead to the knees

Inhale and release as above

Repeat this move for 10 counts

Relax in Shavasana for 5 counts

Hug your knees and roll up - sit on the middle of your hips with knees hugged

Put your feet down and get into Malasana

Malasana

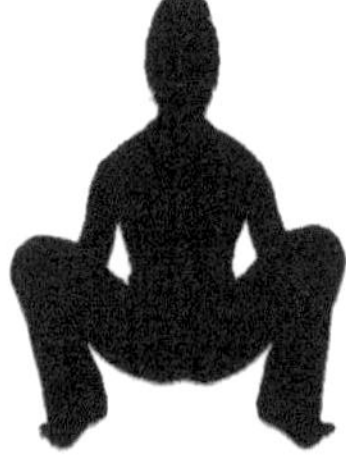

Place legs outside of hips and point toes slightly out

Press down and drop your hip as far down as comfortable

See that the knees point in the direction as the toes. If your hips are tight the knees might turn inwards. Therefore, listen to your body and do not try to exceed your limits

If your heels lift up its fine, if you can, try to keep them down but do not force them

Once down and comfortable, press palms together near the chest

Keep lengthening your spine

Widen your knees with your elbows to open up the hips more

If your heels are close to touching the mat, widen your stance to see if they touch

Stay in the pose for 5 to 8 counts and slowly raise up for standing forward bend

Standing forward bend

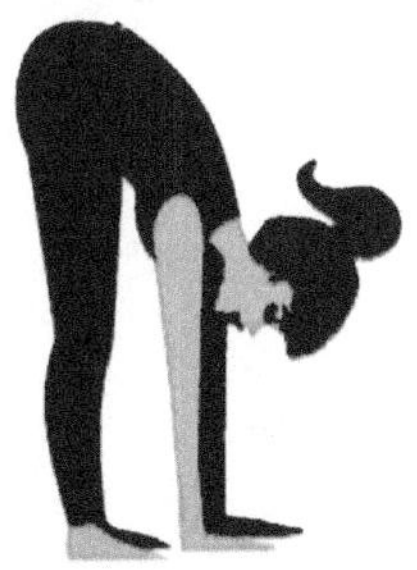

Lift your hips up from Malasana and straighten your legs (try to get into each pose without taking support 'if possible')

Bend from the hips and keep hips in line with the heels

Shoulders away from the ears (by rotating the shoulders outward)

Distribute weight equally on four corners of your feet

Open the chest by drawing the shoulder blades down towards the spine

Ensure to keep a straight back

As you bend your torso engage your core, elongate neck in line with the spine and bring your chest to thighs

The crown of your head faces the mat

Reach for your ankles or your shin or cup your fingers and place the tips on the mat

You can bend your knees slightly and hold onto your shins to lessen the stretch

Raise up in tadasana and get back in a supine position as explained below -

Extend the left leg behind and put the left knee onto the mat

Extend the right leg and put the right knee alongside the left knee

Stand on your knees

(reminding once more to try and practice the above moves without taking any support)

Fold legs and sit on one side of your hip and immediately lower the back onto the mat and raise legs up 90 degrees angle to the torso

Single straight leg stretches

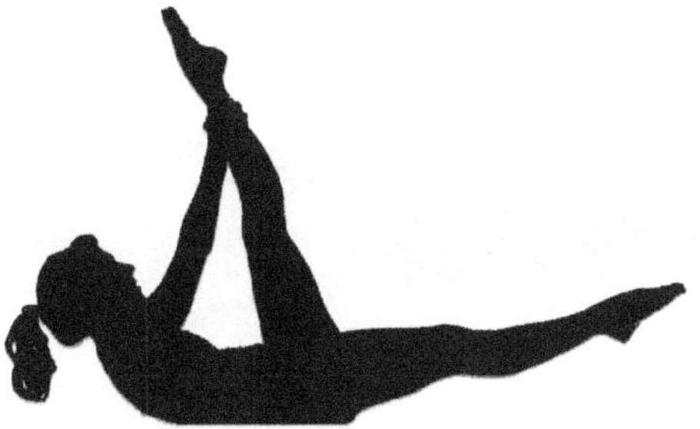

Hold the left ankle with both hands and lower the right leg down up to 45 degrees angle (if possible lower it all the way to the mat and press it into the ground)

Do not arch the lower back and keep lower back pressing towards the mat

Pulse the left leg towards the chest twice and scissor-switch the legs - the left leg comes down and the right leg simultaneously rises up. Hold the right ankle with both the hands

Pulse the right leg twice and scissor-switch the legs again

Repeat the above movements for 10 counts each leg

Rest in Shavasana

Mat criss-cross

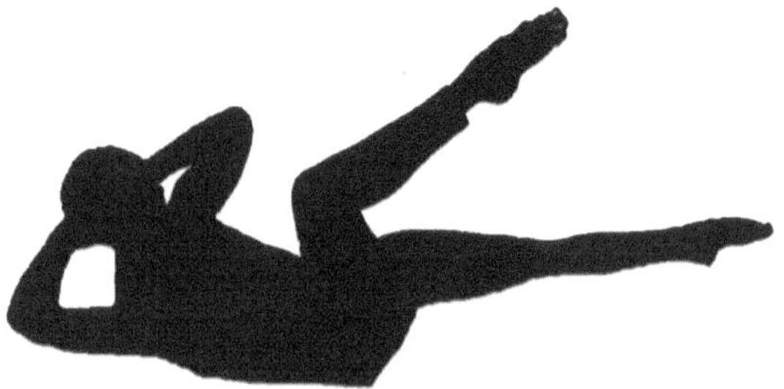

Target the obliques in this move - tone and strengthen them

Bring legs to tabletop position

Raise head neck shoulders till the tip of the shoulder blades

Interlace fingers and place them behind the head as a support for the skull

The elbows remain wide

Keeping pelvis neutral, exhale and pulling abs in deep, extend your right leg long

Simultaneously rotate your torso towards the bent left leg knee such that the right elbow touches the left knee

Inhale and switch legs

Exhale and now extend the left leg long

Simultaneously rotate torso towards the bent right leg such that the left elbow touches the right knee

Switching legs, repeat this move for 10 counts each side

Relax in Shavasana

One leg Teaser

Let's prepare for the Full Teaser

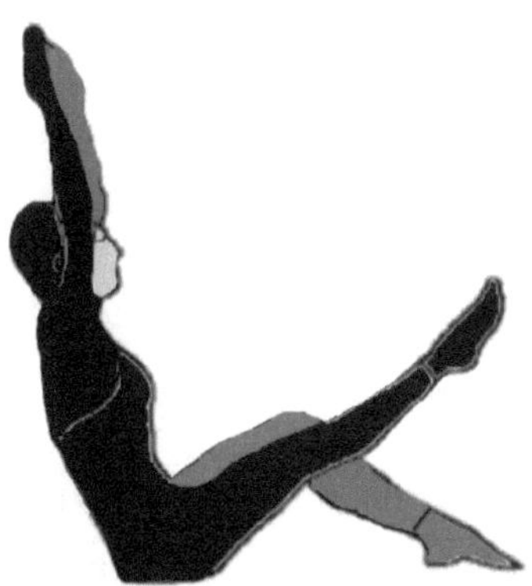

Lie down on your back with a neutral spine

Fold your leg 45-degree angle and feet are flat on the mat

Keep the arms at your sides with palms facing up

Relax your shoulders, drop your ribs back and open up your chest

The legs remain parallel to each other

Inhale and extend the right leg forward keeping the knees at the same height

Simultaneously, slowly raise arms overhead beside the ears and gently roll your upper back off the mat

Your back forms a slight C-curve

The left foot remains flat on the mat

Bring arms forward to reach your knee first, then your ankles and then the sky

Exhale and gently extend arms behind you as you roll down on the mat

Immediately inhale and roll up, bringing arms forward the same way - to reach your knee first, then your ankles and then the sky

Let the flow of rolling up and down be very smooth. Don't jerk and use your abs to come up and go down

Do 10 repetitions

Lie down on your back, relax and maintain a neutral spine and pelvis

Arms are lying on the mat beside you with collar bones broad

Double leg Teaser

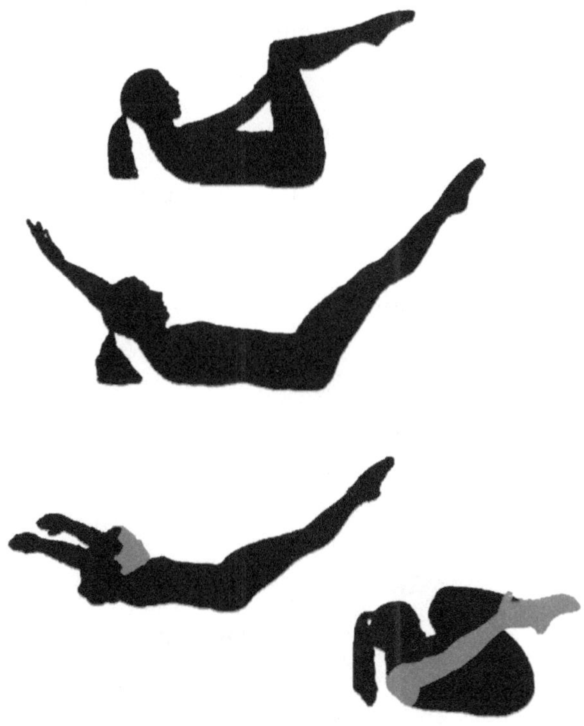

Raise the right leg to tabletop and then the other leg

Inhale and relax the body

Exhale and lift the head neck shoulders up till the tip of the shoulder blades. The arms reach for the ankles or the shins

You can also bring both knees in toward your chest. Curling your head up extend hands and place them on your knees

Inhale and make a circle of your arms and reach the arms overhead. Straighten your leg as much as you can, keeping the spine neutral

Exhale and circle your arms out and around your knees; and pull the knees towards your chest

Do 8 to 10 repetitions

Relax in Shavasana

Konasana

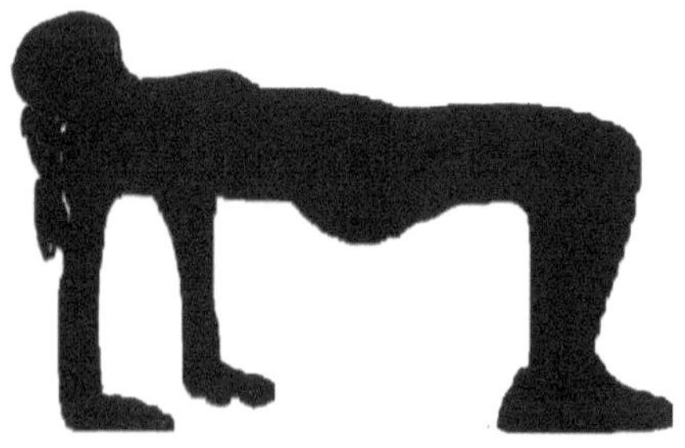

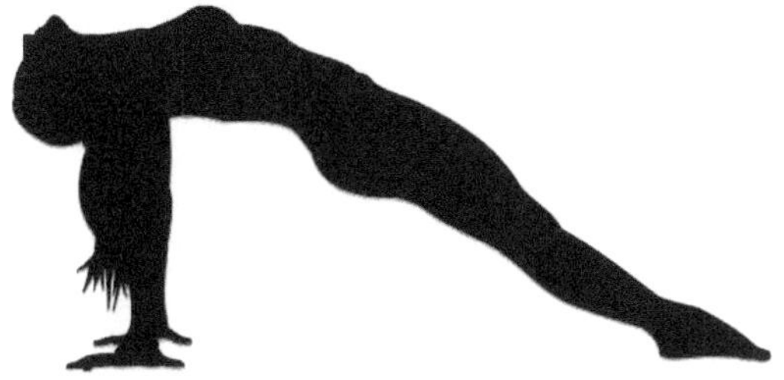

Pressing elbows gently, sit up in long sitting with hands several inches behind the hips and fingers pointing forward

Fold legs with knees facing the roof and feet flat on the mat

Press your palms and inner feet and raise your hips up until your back and torso are almost parallel to the mat and hands and shins somewhat perpendicular to the mat

The shoulders are in one line with the wrists

You are now in a reverse tabletop position

Maintain the height of hips and straighten one leg at a time

Engage your core, keep your hips soft and lift hips more. Keep feet pressing down onto the mat

Lift up the chest to the sky

Keeping neck soft, drop the head back

Relax for 10 counts

To come out of the pose, you can come to the tabletop pose by bending back the legs one after the other

Slowly put hips down, lower you back onto the mat and relax in Shavasana

Hug your knees and roll up

Put the feet down on the mat and without any support get into Malasana

From Malasana, as explained earlier, get into a standing forward bend

Micro bend your knees, cross your palms, make a nice circle of arms and get into tadasana

Seated knee tucks

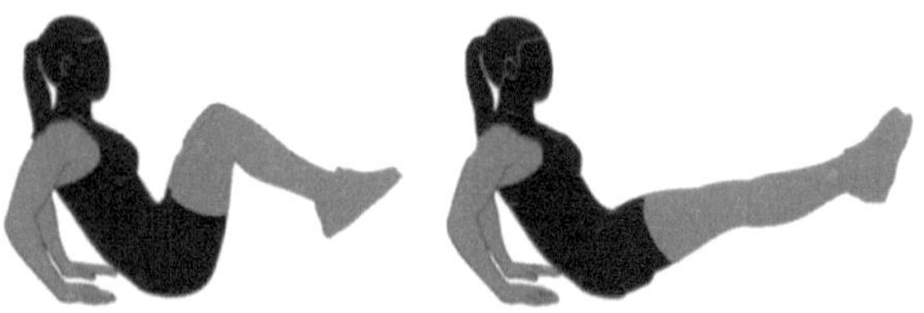

Leaves every muscle in your core with fire
Slowly raise your torso up putting slight weight on your forearms and elbows

Place your palms about one to two inches behind your back. Fingers are facing forward

Legs folded with knees facing up. Your feet are on the ground

Inhale and lift your feet off the mat and extend it forward and simultaneously lower your body backward

Your feet should not touch the ground

Exhale and with total control pull your legs back to your chest without touching the ground

Inhale and again extend legs forward pushing body backward

Repeat 15 to 20 repetitions

You can also do it with one leg at a time - switching it up by alternating knees

Relax in Shavasana

Roll-ups pilates

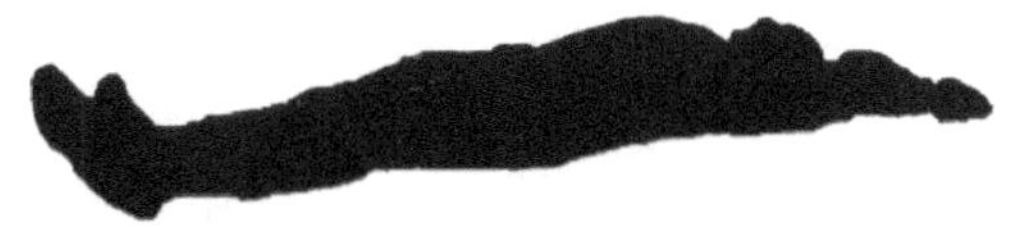

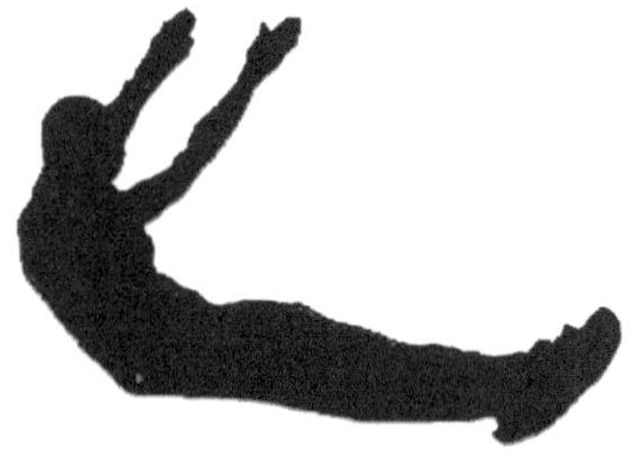

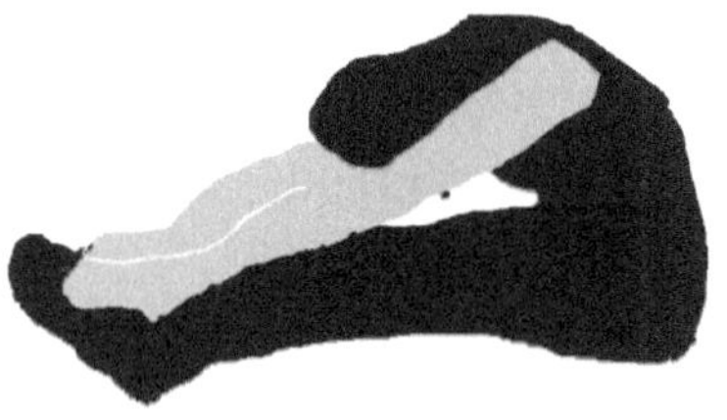

Engage more muscle fibres in this exercise when compared to the other core exercises

Extend arms overhead and keep the legs long and flex your feet

Inhale and lift your arms and curl your chin and chest forward

Exhale, engage your abs, and roll up the entire torso and reach up the toes

Inhale and start the rollback of the spine one vertebra at a time

Exhale once the arms reach back overhead and the base of the middle back touches the mat

Inhale and roll up again and repeat the exercise for 8 to 10 repetitions

Let the movements be slow and gentle, using the abs to lift and lower the torso

Pull abdominals down into a deep scoop as you curl up and curl down

Keep the lower legs down and the toes flexed

If you experience legs popping up then roll up only as much as you can, or bring your knees up with feet on the mat and the results will still be awesome

Relax in Shavasana

Pilates Saw

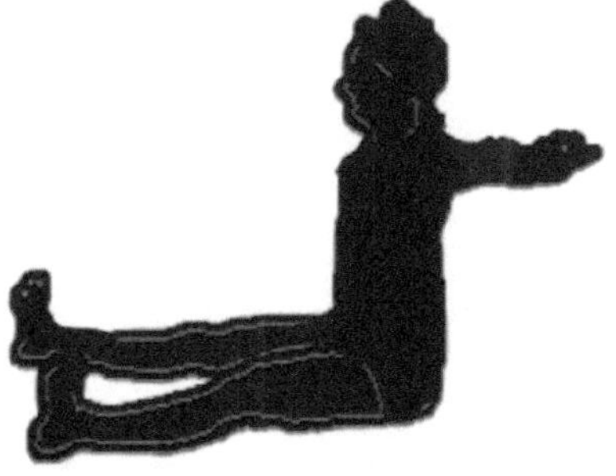

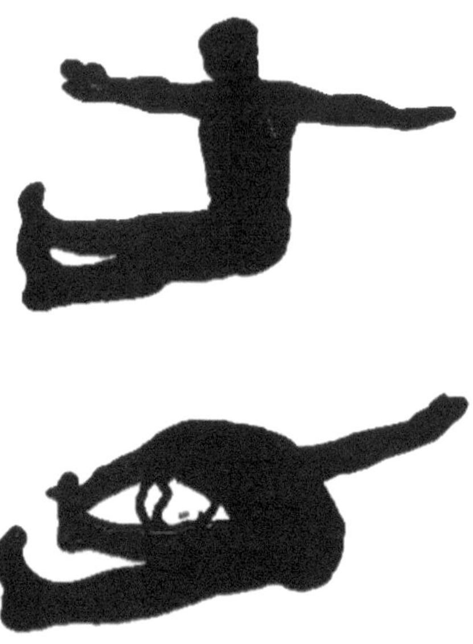

Pressing forearms and elbows gently raise torso and sit up with legs apart and feet flexed

Stretch your arms out to the sides

Twist your upper body to the right side and reach the left hand to the outside of the right ankle and reach the right arm back

You can either gaze at the right arm or gaze down onto the right knee

Repeat on the other side

Total 10 repetitions on each side

Relax in Shavasana

Shoulder bridge series

Let's burn the cellulite on the hamstrings and the butt

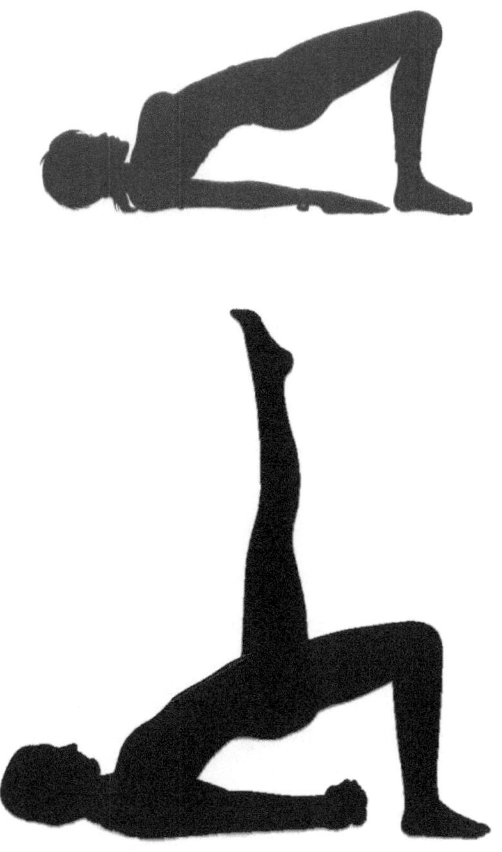

Bridge

Fold your legs at the knees with your feet flat on the mat and hip-distance away

Stack your knees and heels. The toes point forward

Keep your shoulders sliding from the ears to avoid neck/shoulder tensions

Bring the arms under the hips, press the elbows lightly and raise your chest and head off the mat

Gently bring the crown of your head on the mat, keeping your toes pointed

Ensure there is no pressure on your head and neck

Stay in the pose for 5 counts

Repeat 4 rounds

Release torso and head to the mat

Single leg bridge

Inhale and lift right leg up as you raise your hips up

Ensure that the left toes keep pointing forward and not sideways as you lift one leg up

Also, keep shoulders away from the ears

Engage your abs and curl your tailbone towards the ceiling

Exhale and lift hips up completely to make a diagonal line with the shoulders

If you have tight hamstrings (inner thighs) you can bend the lifted leg

The sole of the right foot faces the roof

Remain in the pose for 2 counts, exhale and come down

Do four repetitions

Repeat with the left leg

Relax in Shavasana

Leg rotation in bridge pose

Same as above till you raise the right leg up

Rotate the right leg clockwise - keep circles small like the big toe is drawing small circles (the size of a ping pong ball)

10 rotations clockwise and 10 rotations anti-clockwise

Relax in Shavasana

Rolling like a ball

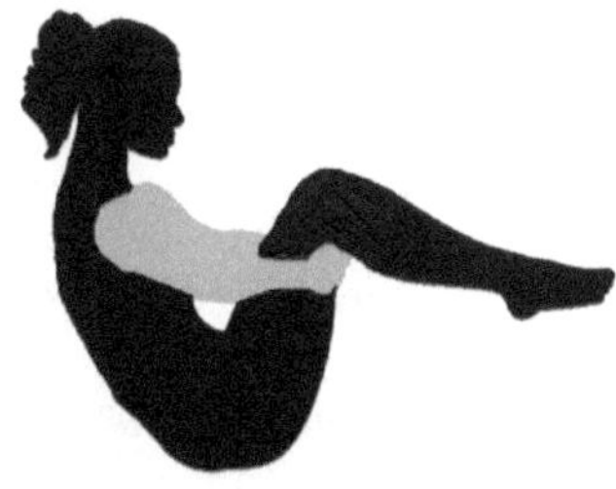

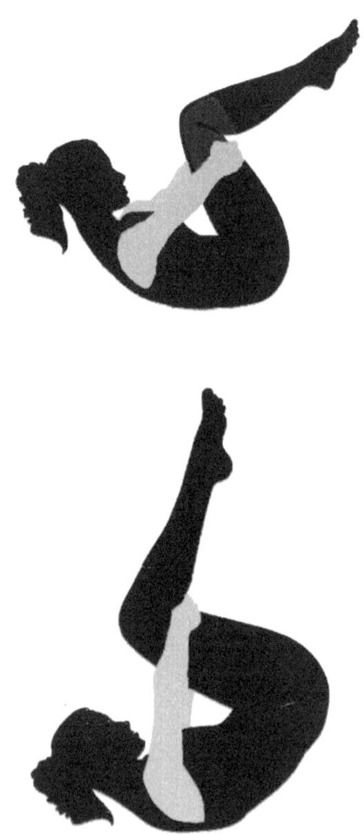

Looks simple but is deceptively tough

Sit up in a long sitting pose

Fold your legs bringing your knees to the chest and hold your inner thighs as shown in the pic

Rollback a little till you are balancing on your tailbone

Lift feet and toes slightly off the mat

Inhale and tilt backward, curling your body like a ball, roll down onto your shoulder blades

Exhale and immediately roll up engaging your abdomen. No effort on the lower back and all effort on your abs to roll back up into your sitting balancing pose

The flow from rolling down onto the mat and back up should be extremely smooth and without any jerks

The neck and shoulders remain silent and relaxed

Continue for 6 to 8 repetitions, coordinating movement with the breath

Relax in Shavasana

With this ends our second module

The instructions above for each exercise is given keeping in mind the beginner's level. If you are a pilates or yoga pro and not a beginner then you can bring in some challenges, like:

Perform each move longer than the time listed

If you are an advanced practitioner then focus on the correct form, coordinate movements perfectly with the breath, and I can guarantee that you will feel the burn in every muscle

You can also use 1 to 2 kgs of dumbbells for an added challenge

With this, we finish our yogalates workout, and I hope the experience of changing pace and trying something new was FUN!

Applying the quote, 'variety is the spice of life' to our exercise routine, brings in different benefits to the table. A well-rounded fitness program, along with guaranteed weight loss, helps us gain strength, cardiovascular endurance, flexibility, agility, balance, grace, ease and much more

If your body has had a good workout then there are chances of muscles getting sore. A little soreness is good but not to the extent that you are incapable of doing your day to day chores like taking care of your family or going to work, etc. The soreness should go away within 2 to 3 days, and the chances of experiencing it again also reduced

Wish you all the best on your journey to achieve your fitness goals; keep in mind these important points to support your body for future workouts:

Help muscles recover

Do not over stress your muscles

Sleep well

Hydrate yourselves well

Eat nutritious food

Stay relaxed always

CHAPTER 7

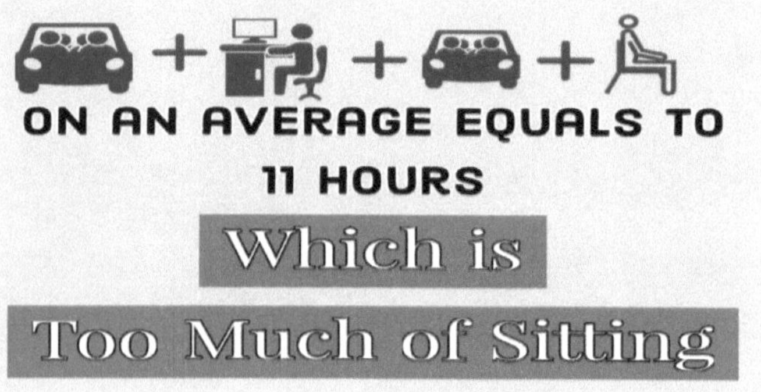

7. DO YOU SUFFER FROM SITTING DISEASE?

Me: Do you suffer from sitting disease?

You: Yes

Me:

"For people who sit most of the day, their risk of heart attack is same as that of smoking" ~Martha Grogan cardiologist Mayo clinic.

Do you know that if you sit for more than 23 hours a week, you are more likely to die of heart disease? Sedentary (overall inactivity or prolonged sitting) lifestyle statistic says that 20% of all deaths of people 35years and older are attributed to a lack of physical activity

You: Its extremely scary

Me: Yes, it is. So, get Moving Today

You: But how? My job requires me to sit all the time be it on the roads or at the desk.

Me: Yes, it is not only our desk-bound jobs that require prolonged sitting but today we sit for almost everything, may it be traveling, waiting, eating, studying and relaxing.

Sitting disease is the new health epidemic and it is the result of sedentary lifestyles and over sitting.

One simple test - after sitting for 30 minutes, stand up and try to touch your toes. Is the back of your legs tight? If yes then it is because of sitting too much

You: But then I am physically fit and exercise regularly for 60 minutes every day?

Me: Healthy living requires movement and not just exercise. The Journal of Medicine and Science in Sports and Exercise says that people who are physically fit are also at risk of sitting disease. Even if you exercise for an hour, the rest of the 8 to 9 hours you still sit and you remain at a risk from suffering from sitting disease.

Therefore, it has to be a whole day approach to movement.

You: Can you help?

Me: You have to help yourself in a very simple way. Read On

The problem with chair sitting is, the body being too smart adapts to the position that you have been the most, and, when you get up after uninterrupted sitting, the body does not unfold neatly and instead develops some tight and sticky spots. The body then has to make all sorts of compensation to stand straight. These compensations overtime lead to pains, injuries, and discomforts.

The number of hours you sit (i.e. if you slouch and sit on the tailbone) - the same number of hours:

- Your hips and knees remain in a static position.

- The quads (the upper thigh) and the glutes. (the group of three muscles that make up your buttocks) are stretched.

- The hamstrings (the inner thigh muscles) are shortened. The upper attachment of the quads is shortened and the portion of the quads that cross the knee is shortened too.

All this results in tight hips, tighter leg muscles and a tight lower back.

What if you have the habit of sitting on your toes? Unknowingly you are tightening the: -

- Top of your toes to the top of the feet.

- The Achilles tendons (the tough band of fibrous tissues connecting the calf muscles to the heel bone).

- The calf muscles.

- The back of the knee.

- The groins.

- The back.

Consistently sitting with a poor posture affects your spine health too - such as compressing the discs in the spine leading to premature degeneration of the discs.

Uninterrupted sitting for as little as 30 minutes results in a chain reaction that includes inflammation, poor circulation, higher risk to obesity, certain cancers, type 2 diabetes, and cardiovascular diseases.

Your core becomes weak over time and you develop pain and stiffness in the neck and shoulders too.

Q. What should be the ergonomic posture while you sit?

Ans. Sit with shoulder blades pulled back, neck relaxed, elbows by your side and maintain a neutral spine.

Without getting into too much of facts on the basics of sitting and the ill effects of uninterrupted sitting, let us understand the antidote to sitting disease and how to fit movement into our day.

If you are entrapped in a desk-bound day, 20 minutes of stretching, twisting, and bending can be profound. Now, if you say you cannot take out time for this (due to workload), I will say that this shall make you more productive in the last two hours of the day and acts as an antidote when your steam is low.

To start with:

You reach office after an hour or two of car travel, and that has already frayed your nerves. As you do not have an option other than this, I would say that make the commuting as stress-free as possible.

1. Listen to an audiobook, a playlist (sing along if possible).

2. Listen to a podcast.

3. Meditate and keep telling yourself that the others are also in the same situation as yours.

4. Wear comfortable clothes and comfortable shoes.

Once you reach office, take the stairs instead of the elevator to get your:-

- Leg pumping
- Exercise your bones and muscles and

- Produce 'happy hormones'

This lowers the risk of developing type 2 diabetes, heart diseases, and osteoporosis. The best part is you also burn calories and that too 2 to 3 times more than brisk walking.

After the first hour of work, do these:

Half squats, knee raises and calf raises, 20 seconds each and 3 repetitions of each. This comes to around 3 minutes (only)

Half squats

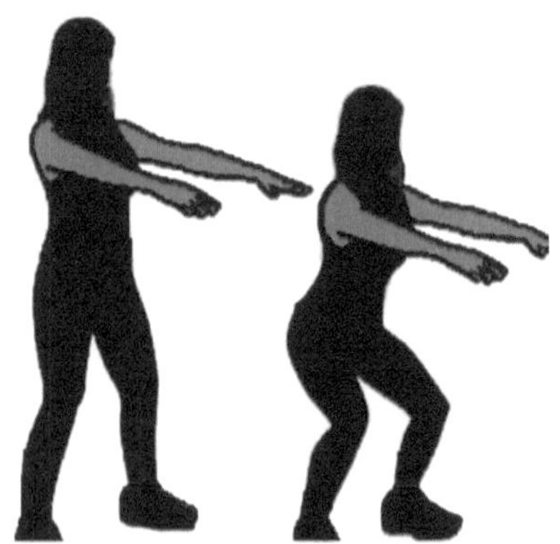

1. Stand straight with legs wide.
2. Bend your legs and push your butt back 45

degrees angle. Just go halfway and not a full
   sit.

3. As you bend down, extend arms straight in front
    of you.

4. Pause for 20 counts and slowly raise up back
    pushing through your heels.

5. Keep your knees soft and do not lock them.

6. Repeat 3 times.

Knee raises

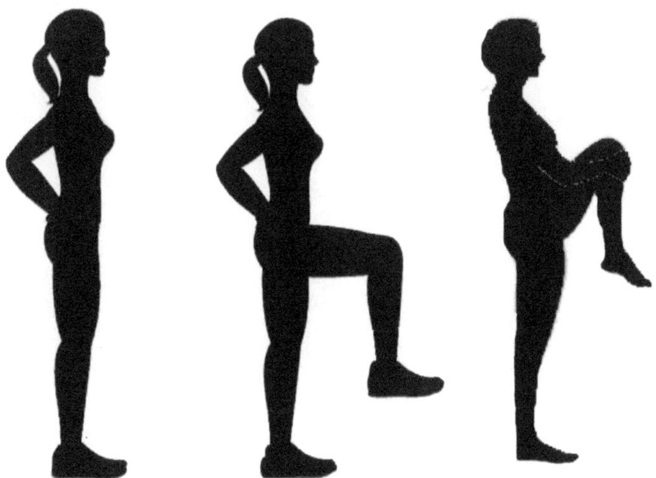

1. Stand with legs apart, hip-distance.

2. Arms holding both sides of the waist.

3. Raise the right leg up with the leg bent at the knee.

4. Raise the right knee till the quads (the inner thigh) is parallel to the mat.

5. Hold for 10 counts.

6. If balance is a problem you can hold your leg as shown in the picture above.

7. Lower the right leg back and bring the right feet flat on the mat.

8. Repeat 3 times.

9. Repeat the same with the left leg - 3 repetitions.

Calf raises

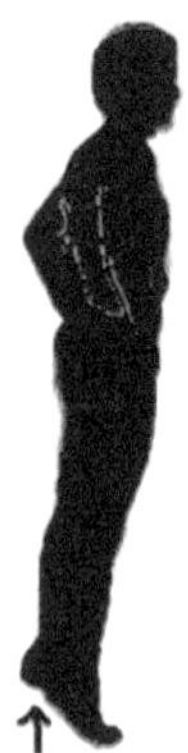

1. Stand straight with feet a little apart.

2. Arms holding the sides of your waist.

3. Push through the balls of your feet and raise your heels.

4. Keep raising heels slowly till you stand on your toes.

5. Hold for 20 counts.

6. Slowly lower back till feet are flat on the mat.

7. Repeat 3 times.

Add to these:

Shoulder rotations

Raise your left shoulder to the ear, move it backward, downwards and around in one continuous motion. This completes one round. Repeat the move 5 times and switch directions.

Repeat the same with the other shoulder.

The back, chest, abs and the rest of the body should remain silent and only the shoulders should move.

This should take 10 seconds.

Arm stretch

Extend your arms to your sides in line with shoulders.
Make a fist with your thumb out.

Fold your forearm so that it forms a 90-degree angle with the upper arm.

The upper arm should be parallel to the mat.

Fold your forearm down from the elbow, until the front side of your forearm is parallel to the mat.

Maintain the 90-degree angle between the forearm and the upper arm.

Raise the forearm back to position.

Repeat 5 times.

This takes around 10 seconds.

The upper arms, shoulders, neck and other parts of the body should remain silent and only the forearm and fist should move.

Neck Exercises

a. Make a fist of your right hand with the thumb in.

   Bring the fist under your chin.

   Inhale and press your chin upwards and pause for two counts (the fist should not move).

   Exhale and press the chin downwards (gently touching the fist) and pause for two counts.

Repeat the same 4 to 5 times.

b. Keeping the neck long and chin raised, inhale and turn the head towards the right. Pause for one count.

Exhale and bring it back to the centre.

Inhale and turn the head towards the left and pause for one count.

Exhale and bring it back to the center.

Repeat the same 3 to 4 times on each side.

c. Hold your left shoulder with your right palm and pull your chin in.

The neck should stay long with your head held upright.

Slowly turn your head towards your left shoulder. The chin should now be parallel to the left shoulder.

Gaze towards your left.

Press the head towards the right shoulder (as if you are trying to pull your right ear towards your right shoulder).

Gently force your ear towards the shoulder.

Gaze up and let the neck sit in this position for 5 counts.

The stretch is felt on the neck muscle on the opposite side.

Repeat the same on the other side, with 4 repetitions on each side.

The a, b, and c of the neck exercises takes on an average 30 seconds

Caution: The exercises above have to be done gently without haste and without any jerks. Do not repeat them for more than 2 times a day...once in the early hours and one in the last activity break.

Results from various research studies recommend 'move 3 minutes for every 30 minutes' therefore, if you can do these simple stretch after every 30 minutes it would be great. If not 30 minutes, I suggest starting with every 60 minutes.

These intermittent bouts of movement will definitely activate your but, legs, arms, core and your back and will also have a positive influence on metabolic factors directly related to the various ailments mentioned above. Some of you might wish to have creative ideas of movement other than just repeating the same sequence of exercises every time. Some of you might feel awkward doing them in the middle of the cubicle with stares from your co-workers. Then take a look at the other activities listed below:

I.   *Walk up and down the stairs for 3 minutes.*

II.   *Do wall push or desk push-ups for 30 seconds, walk 30/30 i.e. walk briskly for 30 seconds followed by a slow and comfortable walk for another 30 seconds - this equals 2 minutes. Finally, repeat the wall/ desk push-ups for the last 30 seconds.*

Desk pushups:

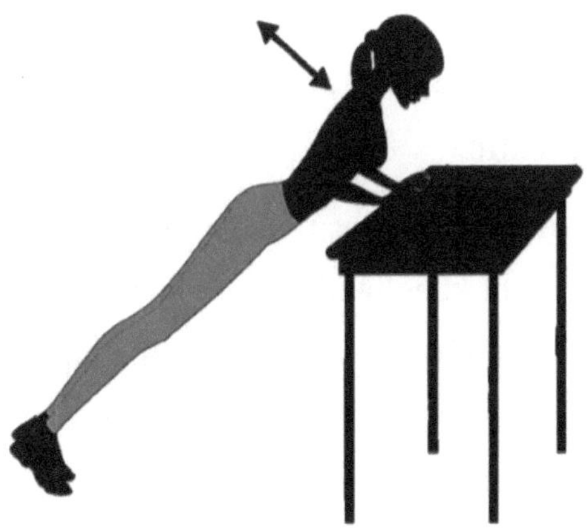

III.   *10 rounds of single-leg deadlifts, standing thigh stretch and windmill jacks.*

Single leg deadlifts:

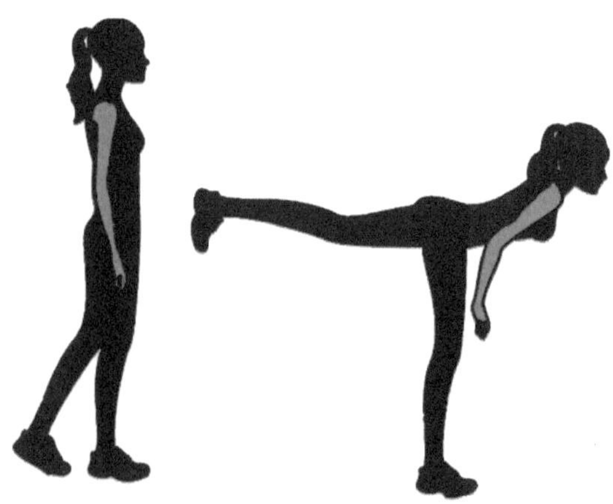

1. Stand with feet together, and stack the hips, knees, and feet.

2. Take the support of the chair or wall with your right arm.

3. Shift weight on the right leg (you can micro bend the right knee) and swing your left leg back till it is straight and in line with the hips and back. Simultaneously, bend down from your hips till your torso is parallel to the mat.

4. Your body now is in a straight line from the bottom of your left foot to the top of your head. Tip your body forward and lower your left arm.

5. Look down with fingers pointing the mat.

Standing thigh stretch:

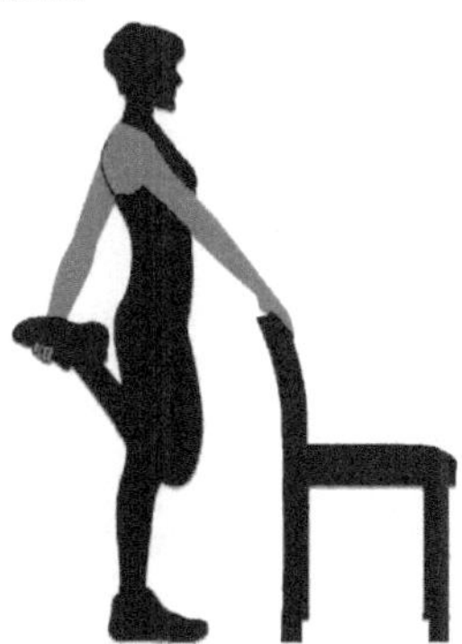

1. Stand straight with your arms by to your sides and feet together.

2. Transfer weight on the left foot.

3. Flex your abs. Bend your right knee and kick your right heel on your right buttock.

4. Grab your right heel with the right arm and let the left arm remain by your side. If you cannot balance then hold the chair with the left arm for support.

5. The chair has to be hip height or higher. This will prevent you from stooping.

6. Keep your knees together. Stack your right knee and right hip.

7. Hold the stretch for 30 seconds.

8. Repeat with the other leg.

Standing windmill stretch

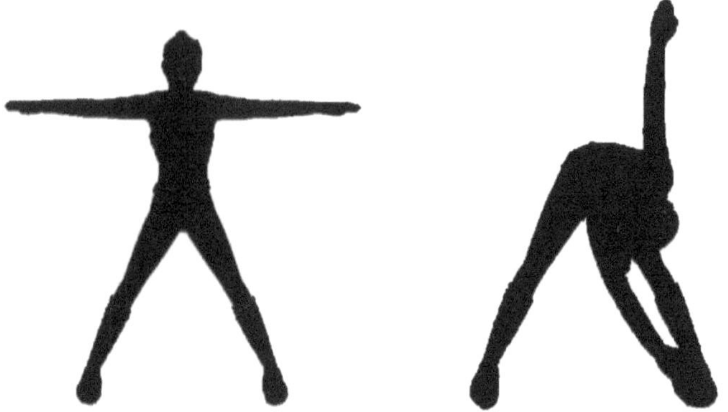

1. In standing position, widen your legs about twice the shoulder-width apart.

2. Bend from the hips and turn your torso towards your right leg.

3. Bring your left arm down either flat on the mat or inside of your right foot and simultaneously lift the right arm as high as possible.

4. Reverse this movement and do it on the left side.

5. Continue on alternate sides for 10 repetitions on each side.

IV. Seated hamstring stretch - 15 seconds each leg and 3 repetitions, overhead triceps stretch - 10 seconds each side and 2 repetitions, shoulder stretch - 10 seconds each side and 2 repetitions, chest stretch 15 seconds and 2 repetitions.

Seated hamstring stretch

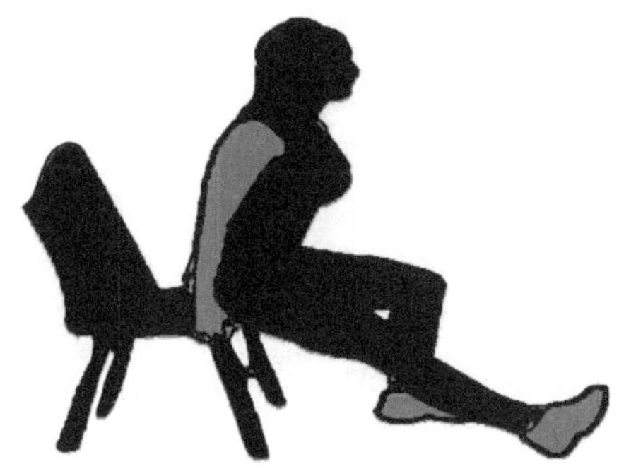

1. Sit on the edge of the chair.

2. Extend right leg forward with the heel on the floor.

3. Flex your abs and straighten up, and push your navel towards the thighs.

4. Keep your body straight and avoid leaning the trunk forward.

5. Hold the stretch for 20 seconds.

6. Repeat with the other leg.

Overhead tricep stretch

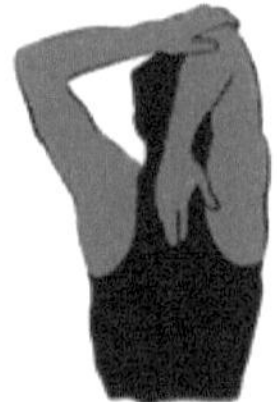

1. Raise your right arm straight up to the roof and bend at the elbow to bring the palm towards the center of your shoulders, and rest the fingers along the spine.

2. With your left arm, hold your right elbow and push it towards the center and downwards.

3. Hold for 10 seconds and repeat on the other side.

4. You can do this either standing or sitting..

Shoulder stretch

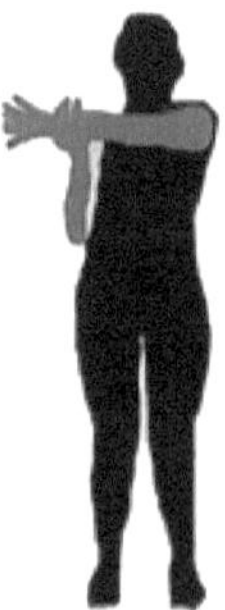

1. Extend the right hand forward and straight, perpendicular to the body.

2. Gently bring it across the body.

3. Extend the left arm diagonal to the body and lock the right arm at the right elbow by folding the left arm 90 degrees angle at the elbow.

4. Press the right arm into the chest and over the left.

Chest stretch

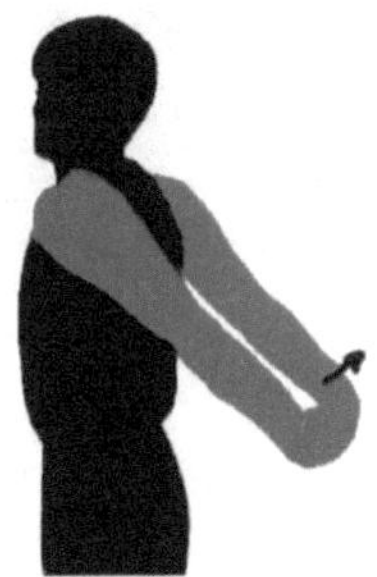

1. Extend both arms back and place the back of the palms on the butt.

2. Interlace fingers near the butt.

3. The back should remain straight.

4. Push your arms upwards and pull the shoulder blades together.

5. Slowly push the interlaced fingers up towards the roof.

6. Hold the pose for 10 seconds and release.

7. Repeat 3 times

V.   Tricep dips 20 counts, chair leg lifts - each leg 10 times, leg swings - each leg 10 times and chair spinal twist - 30 seconds hold each side.

Tricep dips

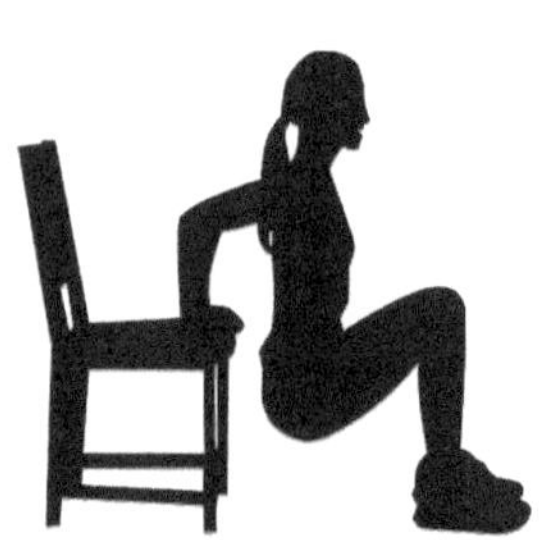

1. Sit at the edge of the chair.

2. Extend the legs with feet hip with apart.

3. Let the heels of the feet touch the ground and toes point upwards.

4. Grip the edge of the chair next to your hips with fingers pointing towards you.

5. Raise chin up and look forward.

6. Gently lift the body up with the support of your arms.

7. Drive the weight into the palms of the hands and the soles of the feet and slide your buttock down.

8. If possible, keep lowering till the elbows reach a 45 to 90-degree angle.

9. Hold for 2 counts.

10. Engaging the biceps to push the body back up to the start position

11. Begin with 5 to 6 repetitions and then slowly increase the count to 10 and then 15

Chair leg lifts

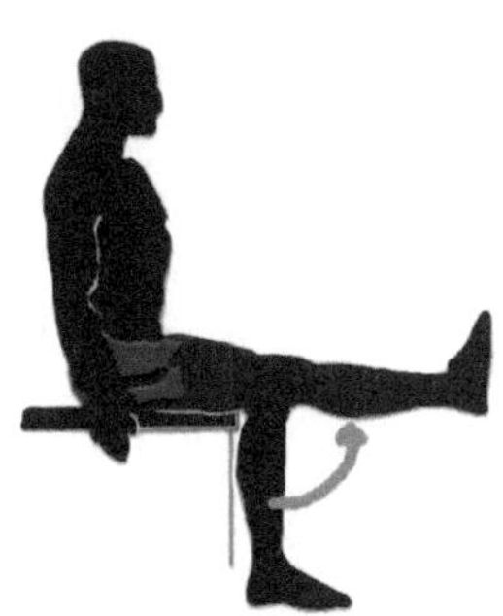

1. Sit on the edge of the chair.

2. Grip the chair on both sides of the hip.

3. Legs are bent and feet are flat on the floor.

4. Swing the right leg and straighten the leg.

5. Flex your toes and squeeze your upper thigh muscles.

6. Keep your body straight throughout.

7. Hold for 5 seconds and bring the leg back to start position.

8. Repeat 10 times and switch sides.

Chair leg swings

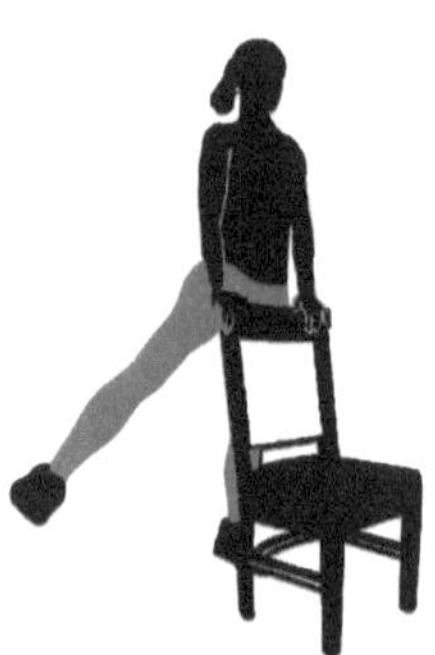

1. Stand up and hold your chair.

2. Keep the feet together or a little away.

3. Engage your abs and lift up the right leg.

4. Swing it up straight as far as you can without moving your torso.

5. Bring the leg back down.

6. Swing up again and repeat this 10 times.

7. Switch legs.

Chair spinal twist

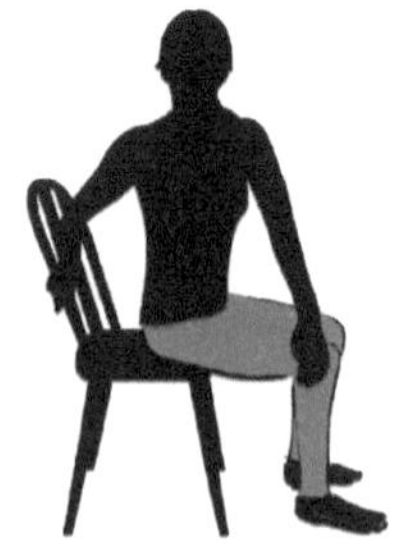

1. Sit at the edge of the chair.

2. The knees should be parallel to each other and right above the ankles.

3. Feet flat on the floor.

4. Keep your spine straight, chin raised and lined up with the middle of the chest.

5. Lengthen the back of the waist, pull abs in towards the spine, gently press hips and twist from your navel onto the right side.

6. Simultaneously bring the left arm towards the right side and hold the sides of the right knee, and hold the right edge of the chair with the right arm (fold the right arm at the elbow)

Let's now get to the eyes and neck, that gets tired staring at the screen for the whole day

Your eyes affect how your neck feels.

Why?

Because 6 muscles behind your eyes connect to your neck!

Also, the Fascia runs from the head over the neck and down to the feet.

Therefore, massaging the top of your head often has a tremendously positive effect on the feeling of the neck.

Give this short sequence a go and feel the difference.

Build it into your daily routine at the office!

Eye massage:

Massage between eyes and nose:

Using your index finger gently press and release (without lifting up your finger) the point right above the inner corner of the eye where the eyelid begins. Do this for 30 seconds.

Massage area between eyes and eyebrows

Using the front side of your thumb, the thumb pointing towards the nose, gently massage the area between the eyes and eyebrows for 30 seconds. The movement of the thumb is towards the nose.

Massage your temples

Using your middle finger and using an up and down motion, massage the hollow part in the temples on both sides of the face. Do this for 30 seconds.

Massage the top of the head:

Using 3 fingers of both arms, start massaging from the back of the head just above the base of the skull making small circles (clockwise) with your fingers.

Keep a distance of 1 to 2 inches and repeat this till you reach the front of the head above the forehead. Repeat this 3 times.

Studies show that computer users blink less and this leads to drying of the eyes. So keep blinking!

Take an activity break every hour and set your timer for each hour and do one of them when the timer goes off.

Download these apps on your pc or on your mobile (pc is recommended) and add years to your life.

- *STAND UP! THE WORK BREAK TIMER APP on the Apple store for iPhone and iPad*

- *BIG STRETCH REMINDER for Windows*

- *STAND for Mac*

"To me, if life boils down to one thing, it's movement. To live is to keep moving." – **Jerry Seinfeld**

The body thrives on movement, because movement signals the body that things are all ok and puts it in a lesser threat. If movement was not in your list till now, then seek for it and gradually work towards it, and I guarantee that you will never ever be sick of sitting!

All the best for a healthy and happier life

EPILOGUE

8. GET GOING

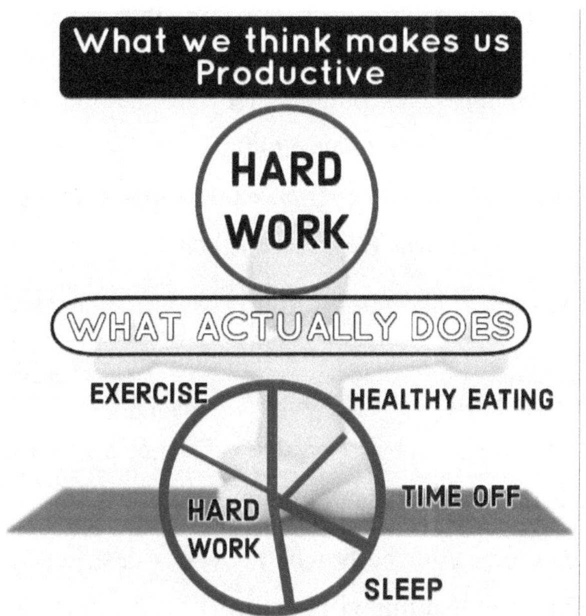

Ask anyone what the secret of productivity is, and the immediate answer would be 'Hard Work'

Right?

No! This is what we think makes us more productive, but what actually does is self-care and self-love.

Why?

'Because 'you cannot give the best of you from what is left of you!'

The obsession with the so-called 'hard work' practically ruins our productivity. In this fast and frenetic life of ours, we are constantly dealing with the invariable stream of messages pinging our systems and our cell phones. We have a never-ending to-do list and all this leads to depletion of energy, exhaustion, burn out and the well runs down. We have to fill ourselves back again.

If a yes, then take out 20 to 30 minutes every day and workout for your physical, mental and emotional wellness. Take some time out for yourself, focus on healthy eating and manage to get proper sleep. Do not forget to take breaks in between your work hours.

Give care to your body when it wants destruction and that is when healing will begin.

Before we say goodbye, if you have enjoyed reading this book meet me in my next book on a spectrum of women's health issues. The book deals with the woman's body being a complex entity, and the factors that can go wrong because of her ability to bear children, and her monthly cycle. How this takes her on a roller coaster of hormonal changes, hormonal imbalance every month from puberty to menopause, and how YOGA without any drama can help women and girls take charge of their body and maximize their personal health and fitness.